DYNAMIC HEALING

A Practitioner's Guide to Reiki Applications

MARINA LANDO & VALERIE REMHOFF

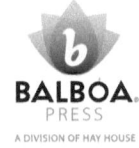

BALBOA.
PRESS

A DIVISION OF HAY HOUSE

Balboa Press books may be ordered through booksellers or by contacting:

Balboa Press
A Division of Hay House
1663 Liberty Drive
Bloomington, IN 47403
www.balboapress.com
1 (877) 407-4847

Because of the dynamic nature of the Internet, any web addresses or links contained in this book may have changed since publication and may no longer be valid. The views expressed in this work are solely those of the author and do not necessarily reflect the views of the publisher, and the publisher hereby disclaims any responsibility for them.

The author of this book does not dispense medical advice or prescribe the use of any technique as a form of treatment for physical, emotional, or medical problems without the advice of a physician, either directly or indirectly. The intent of the author is only to offer information of a general nature to help you in your quest for emotional and spiritual well-being. In the event you use any of the information in this book for yourself, which is your constitutional right, the author and the publisher assume no responsibility for your actions.

Any people depicted in stock imagery provided by Thinkstock are models, and such images are being used for illustrative purposes only.
Certain stock imagery © Thinkstock.

Print information available on the last page.

ISBN: 978-1-5043-3804-2 (sc)
ISBN: 978-1-5043-3806-6 (hc)
ISBN: 978-1-5043-3805-9 (e)

Library of Congress Control Number: 2015912400

Balboa Press rev. date: 12/01/2015

Praise for *Dynamic Healing*

I met Valerie when she became active supporting our Touch for Health (TFH) board of directors, and I was very encouraged by her youthful spirit and positive vision for the work. With this book, she brings a wealth of practical, hands-on tools that will undoubtedly bring greater physical comfort, emotional peace, health and function, and joy and satisfaction in life to many people who practice and receive these techniques. I am delighted to see that she has incorporated a few simple but very powerful tools from TFH/ Energy Kinesiology to enhance and expand the procedures and benefits of the Reiki work presented in this book. Though many of the techniques are intended for experienced Reiki practitioners, the Stress Release protocol, which we call ESR (emotional stress release), is a powerful tool in the hands of the practitioner but also a very accessible technique that anyone can learn and apply from her succinct description, in the educational kinesiology tradition. This book is a valuable testimony and resource for the power that human beings have in their hands, and our ability to support each other through human touch.

Matthew Thie, coauthor *TFH Pocketbook with Chinese 5 Element Metaphors* (2003); *Touch for Health: The Complete Edition* (2005).

This clearly written and illustrated guide is sure to benefit any Reiki practitioner and help take your practice to the next level. Its step-by-step instructions and synthesis of techniques will wonderfully enhance your therapeutic toolkit.

Debra Greene, PhD, author of *Endless Energy*

Marina Lando is the consummate professional in scope and understanding of her work. A woman of integrity and honesty, she brings these characteristics to any endeavor and certainly to her writing with her coauthor Valerie Remhoff in their book *Dynamic Healing.* You'll want to read and use this wonderful approach to living healthfully.

Dr. Natalie L. Winters, psychologist, psychodramatist (TEP), hypnotherapist, and author of *Tools for Happiness: An Easy Guide to a Joyful Life.*

In gratitude to all my teachers: Stanislava Veleten, Emma and Emmanuil Pinsky, Mark Kivin, Diana Henderson, Gin Brunssen, Natalie Winters, and Andrea Butje. For all your lessons, thank you.

Marina Lando, MS, Reiki master and teacher, aromatherapist

To my husband, who has been my number one champion and supporter through my journey into this beautiful field of energy healing, thank you. You are my rock. I love you! To my children, you are my life's joy. Thank you for giving me the mommy time I needed to finish this book! Thank you to all my teachers who have inspired and guided me, and to my friends, family, and clients who have been eager to try all my new techniques. You all hold a special place in my heart.

Special thanks to my Reiki master, Jane Berrigan, for sharing many of the techniques taught in this book.

Valerie Remhoff, BA, Reiki master teacher, IKC certified Touch for Health instructor/consultant.

CONTENTS

FIGURES

PREFACE

This book was born out of the recognition that although Reiki is taught all over the world and the basics are essentially the same, not every Reiki student learns all the same things. Reiki techniques and training are traditionally passed down from master to student, and the information sometimes gets slightly modified through each iteration. Each master brings his own viewpoints and experience into the mix, and new information is passed to students that is meant to enhance their journey and add to their knowledge. Consequently, there is a growing number of great protocols out there that many Reiki students have not had the opportunity to learn.

During our Reiki exchanges together, the authors of this book realized that although we were both attuned to Usui Reiki, our training and methodologies were very different. Comparing our manuals, we found the fundamentals to be similar, but not much else. After our original Reiki training, we had both continued educating ourselves but had gone in two different directions. Marina studied Ayurveda and learned to incorporate its principals into her healing practice. She also developed new protocols through her work that brought her great results with her clients. Valerie continued to study traditional Chinese and Japanese methodologies and the meridian system. She trained in several schools of kinesiology and through her years of practice, developed some highly effective techniques.

Through our sessions together, we recognized the value and effectiveness of each other's work and wanted to find a way to combine and share our knowledge. We also realized that sometimes Reiki students are unsure how to best use all the information that they have learned. Which of the many techniques at their fingertips should they apply in a given situation? This book endeavors to both expand your repertoire and to provide guidance about when and how to use your skills.

In these pages, you will find a vast array of healing protocols. Some may be familiar to you, and some will be brand new. We encourage you to work with each one to get a feel for its healing benefits. Tools are presented to help you determine the best protocol to use at any given time. It is our sincere hope that you will find this book useful and beneficial for you, your family, your friends, and your clients. We hope it will encourage you to continue to expand your knowledge and improve your skills.

ACKNOWLEDGMENTS

We would like to thank Elaine Bryant of Windmill Photography (windmillphotography.net), whose incredible pictures are the basis for all the diagrams in this book. Your eye for light and detail allowed us to create exactly the shapes and lines we needed to convey our message.

Thank you to Diane Brueckmann for her expert help creating the diagrams. You took our vision and brought our ideas to life.

To our editor, Linda Ann McDonald, thank you for going through the book with a fine-tooth comb and finding all those little things we missed.

We would also like to give a big thank-you to all of our friends, family, and colleagues who read the many versions of this book and gave us their valuable input. We could not have done this without you!

THE BASICS

A short history lesson and an introduction to energy anatomy

The "Short and Sweet" History of Reiki

In the beginning of the twentieth century in Japan, the quest for knowledge and ancient wisdom was surpassed only by the skill and art of natural healing. The energetic healing practices of acupuncture and qigong were inherited from China thousands of years before and had become an integral part of the culture. As in other cultures of the time, energy healing was a way of life, not an alternative. In Japan, life-force energy was called ki. The Chinese called it chi, and in India, it was known as prana. It was during this time that Mikao Usui of Japan discovered a healing method that would eventually be utilized throughout the world. He called his system Reiki.

Mikao Usui was on a quest for enlightenment. He had studied the meditative movement practices of qigong to an advanced level and was a student of Shinto Buddhism. According to legend, he was frustrated by the slow pace of his progress and asked his Buddhist master for help. The answer he received was that he should "die one time." Desperately seeking answers, Usui went to Mount Kurama Yama to practice the *shyu gyo*, a spiritual discipline that includes fasting and meditation for twenty-one days. At the end of the twenty-one days, Usui felt a great energy, became enlightened, and acquired a healing ability, which he called Reiki Ryuhi.

Upon returning home, Usui began using his healing ability on others. After further study in Shinto and Mahayana (Mikkyo) Buddhism techniques, Usui discovered Reiju, an empowerment method now called an attunement, and Hatsurei-ho, a cleansing process for the body, mind, and spirit. Through these methods, he was able to directly transfer his healing ability to his students without the need for lengthy training. The first record of Usui giving Reiju was in Harajuku, Tokyo, in 1922.

One of the few Reiki masters that Usui attuned was Chiryo Hayashi. After Usui's death, Hayashi took over his clinic and continued to use and teach Reiki. In 1938, Hayashi attuned Hawayo Takata to the master level and allowed her to bring Reiki to the United States.

About Reiki Symbols

Reiki symbols are traditionally only given to students with second-degree Reiki training. The symbols and their meanings are not discussed in this book. This book is intended for students who have achieved Reiki level 2 and higher training. Since Reiki is a tradition that is passed down from master to student, symbols may be slightly different from master to master. We will assume that each person reading this book has been attuned to the three basic symbols and can use them with these techniques as necessary. If you have not yet achieved Reiki level 2, there is still much to learn from this book; however, we do recommend taking a level 2 Reiki class in order to fully utilize its contents.

The Importance of Self Care for a Reiki Practitioner

In traditional Eastern medicine, it is believed that working with the energy field and balancing chi is the way to heal the body, mind, and spirit. Chi energy surrounds us, flows through us, and connects us all. It is the universal energy of life that makes all things possible. The Reiki practitioner is the channel or conduit for the chi energy and is therefore the tool by which the healing takes place. For this reason, it is important for the practitioner to be in prime condition in order to perform the most effective energy healing.

Starting over five thousand years ago in both Chinese medicine and Ayurveda (the wellness system of India), and continuing through today, healing practitioners have used chi exercises to stay healthy and balanced. Self-healing practices, such as Reiki, meditation, and the focused movements of qigong, are a few of the many options available to practitioners. The use of these methods helps to maintain the vitality of the practitioner which is extremely important when doing any kind of energy work. Regular use of self-healing practices will help improve clarity and focus, and will increase the practitioner's sensitivity to intuition and energy flow. Clear and balanced energy in the practitioner allows for a stronger flow of chi and a more effective session for the client.

Reiki practitioners should therefore make self-care a high priority. Reiki self-healing, Reiki meditations, and practicing on others are all great ways to increase chi flow and maintain health on a regular basis. Make these healing practices and sessions with other healing practitioners part of your routine. You will feel healthy and energized, and your clients will receive the most beneficial sessions you can give them.

The Basic Anatomy of the Human Energy Field

Human beings are more than just physical bodies. We are surrounded and supported by a dynamic field of energy. This energy field, like the physical body, is comprised of many individual systems that work together to maintain our health. The physical body and the energy field feed, support, and affect one another. In order for the whole person to be healthy and balanced, there must be harmony between the energetic and the physical.

Our emotional and mental state also has a great effect on our health. Eastern systems of medicine recognize that the physical body, energy field, and emotions are all parts of an integrated whole. When a person's body is not functioning optimally, feelings of sadness or frustration may develop. Conversely, when a person is depressed or stressed, physical pain, such as a headache, fatigue, or muscle aches may be experienced. Western (allopathic) medical doctors have also studied how the state of the patient's mind influences the outcome of treatment, and they have come to the same conclusion. Depressed patients are more likely to have complications, and the recovery is often slower. Under the same conditions, a patient with a cheerful disposition recovers faster.[1] Full physical recovery requires emotional and mental healing. Often, this can be facilitated by using energy healing techniques.

Chinese and Japanese healers have traditionally worked mainly with the meridian system and acupuncture points. In India, where Ayurveda has been used for over five thousand years, the *chakras*, *marmas*, and *nadis* are emphasized. Each of these systems make up a part of the anatomy of the human energy field. They work both separately and together to help keep us healthy and functioning to our greatest potential.

The energy systems mentioned above by no means comprise an exhaustive list of the parts of the human energy field. They are, however, the systems on which the Reiki protocols taught in this book will focus. In this chapter, you will find a brief overview of each one.

Overview of Chakras and Marmas

Ayurveda is a five-thousand-year-old wellness system from India with an extensive understanding of a wide range of subjects—from prevention and balancing, to surgery, herbal medicine, and psychology. It is still used by many doctors in India, Europe, and America. According to Ayurveda, there is no separation between the physical and energetic body. A person is made of flesh, bones, and an energy field. Mind, spirit, and body affect each other on a constant basis. Thus, an Ayurvedic doctor studies both physical anatomy and the anatomy of the energy field.

---

[1] P. L. Morris, B. Raphael, and R. G. Robinson. "Clinical Depression Is Associated with Impaired Recovery from Stroke." *The Medical Journal of Australia* 157, vol. 4 (1992): 239–242.

The Ayurvedic energy system includes four parts: chakras, marmas, nadis, and koshas (bodies). There are seven main chakras, between 107 and 200 marma points (depending on the school), seventy-two thousand nadis, and five koshas. It is necessary to have a basic understanding of each of these parts in order to perform some of the Reiki protocols in this book. In this section, we will provide a brief explanation of each one.

Chakras

Chakras are energy vortexes that reflect our physical, spiritual, and emotional state. These reservoirs of consciousness float like flowers in front of the body. The "flowers" have their roots in the spine and grow through the body toward the front. There are seven chakras: root (or base), sacral, solar plexus (or power), heart, throat, third eye, and crown. Each of these chakras is associated with a specific function and provides the energy and information exchange among all living organisms and between living organism and environment. When the chakras are open, there is a balance. Blockages in the chakras can cause disturbances in all levels of consciousness.

The following diagram and chart illustrate the location of the seven chakras and describe their basic attributes.

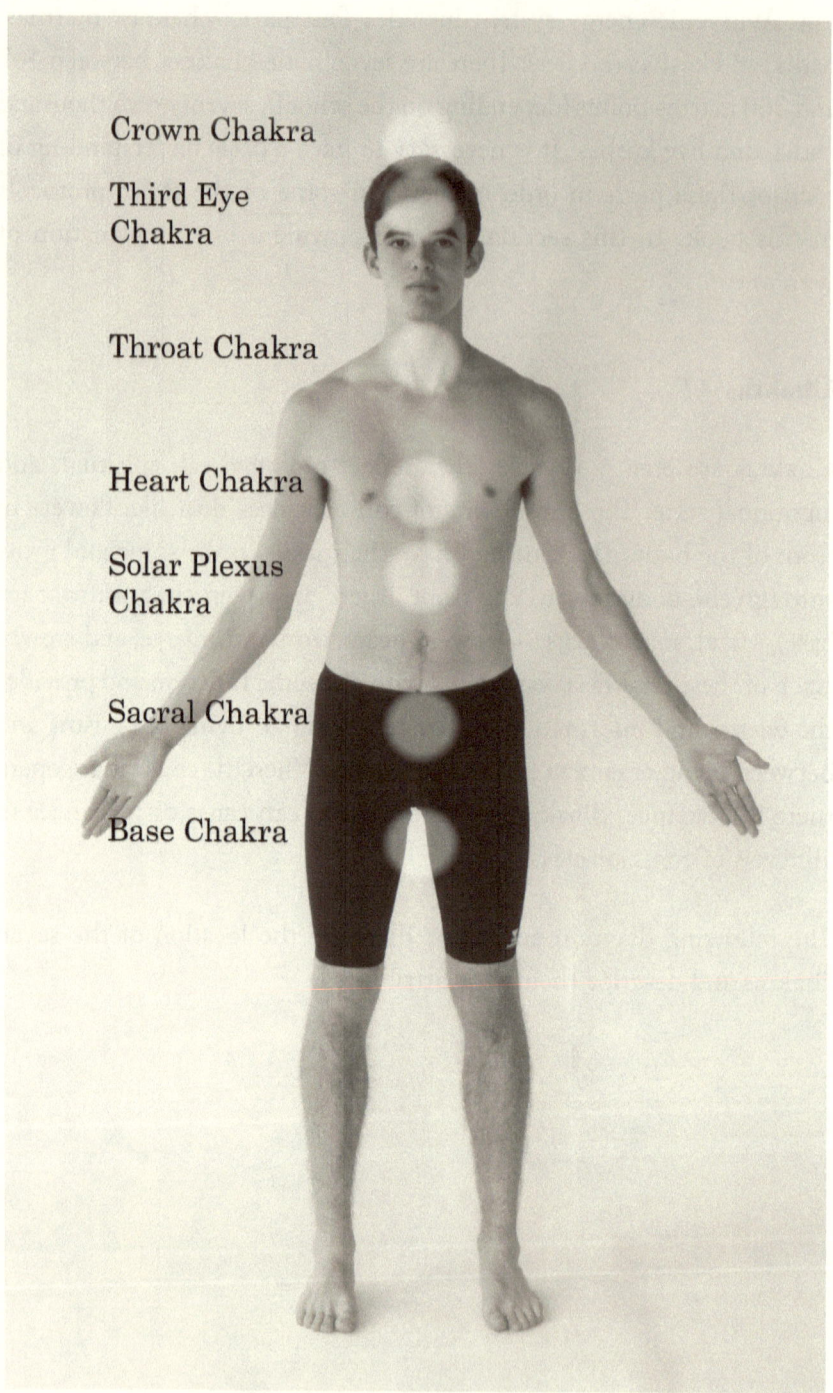

Figure 1: The Chakra System

Chakra	Color	Function	Emotional Imbalance	Physical Imbalance
1 Root/Base	Red	Security, grounding	Stress, insecurity, doubt	Constipation, bone problems, leg pain and injuries
2 Sacral	Orange	Creativity, Sexuality, Control	Stagnation, lack of desire, feeling out of control, jealousy, envy	Infertility, impotence, bladder/kidney problems, lower back problems
3 Solar Plexus/ Power	Yellow	Power, ability to do things	Poor self-esteem, disorder, laziness, inability to start/finish task , anger	Digestive problems
4 Heart	Green	Unconditional Love, compassion	Depression, anxiety, inability to find permanent partner	Heart problems, lung problems
5 Throat	Blue	Self-Expression	Shyness, inability to express feelings/emotions/ ideas	Upper respiratory problems, shoulder pain, neck problems
6 Third Eye	Indigo	Intuition, Acceptance	Inability to accept the reality and predict the outcome	Eye / ear / sinus problems, headaches
7 Crown	Violet	Spirituality / Connection to Divine	Severe depression, suicidal thoughts, inability to learn	Nervous system problems

Figure 2: Chakra Attributes

Nadis

Nadis, are energy channels that allow chi to flow throughout the body. Seventy-two thousand nadis branch from the seventh chakra (crown chakra) and encompass the whole body. There are fourteen principal nadis.

Koshas ("Bodies")

Koshas ("bodies") are the levels of self that make up a whole person. Chi flows through each one, connecting them and helping us maintain our vitality. Ayurveda recognizes five koshas:

- **bliss body** – soul, body of light
- **wisdom body** – the manifestation of the intellect
- **mental body** – personhood
- **breath body** – energy that holds together the physical body
- **physical or food body** – actual physical body, physical self

When the mind is clear, chi flows through all five bodies unobstructed, helping the physical body to function properly. When the mind is foggy, chi stagnates and creates blockages and imbalances that could lead to illness.

We can find an analogy for this in the computer world. Software must work properly to ensure a computer's functionality. When software breaks due to a bad update or a computer virus, this can affect the computer's hardware and cause it to stop working properly. The energy and the physical body are much the same. Issues in the energy field can have a direct effect on physical health.

Marmas

Marma points are located on the surface of the skin. They are described as doorways of consciousness and as golden bolts that connect the energy field with the physical body. Many marma point locations correspond directly with the location of acupuncture points in traditional Chinese medicine. Though marmas are sometimes called "minor chakras" or "secondary chakras," marmas and chakras are actually very different.

Marma points assist the free exchange of chi and information between the physical and energy bodies and can be used to balance physical and emotional disturbances. Reiki is used on marma points to assist the energy flow and to remove the blockages that are affecting the body on all levels: physical, emotional, mental, and spiritual. When the blockage is removed, the chakras become balanced. By evaluating and balancing chakras, trained practitioners can help their clients to improve their emotional and physical states and create positive changes in all aspects of their lives.

Explanation of Meridians

Meridians are energy lines or highways that carry vital energy to all parts of the body. They feed the muscles and organs and provide the energy that keeps us balanced and healthy. Disruption in the flow of the meridians can lead to imbalance and stress on the physical, mental, emotional, or spiritual levels. If meridian imbalances are not corrected, health issues can follow.

There are twelve major meridians that are found bilaterally in the body. These meridians are named for the organs or systems they support and are grouped in sets according to the five elements. The elements are fire, earth, metal, water and wood. Each element is associated with two meridians, one yin (female) and one yang (male), with the exception of

11

the fire element for which there are two yin and two yang meridians. The relationships are as follows:

- **fire** – small intestine, heart, triple warmer, circulation-sex
- **earth** – stomach, spleen
- **metal** – large intestine, lung
- **water** – bladder, kidney
- **wood** – gall bladder, liver

Each major meridian is related to specific muscles of the body, and when energy flow in the meridian is disrupted, those muscles cannot function to their optimal capabilities. This can manifest as pain, postural stress, discomfort, etc. Keeping the energy flow healthy helps to keep the muscles healthy and strong.

The meridians run on a twenty-four-hour cycle, called the horary cycle, where every two hours a different meridian and its associated organ is at its maximum energy and activity. When imbalances occur, it is sometimes noticeable based on this cycle. For example, if someone is waking up every night at the same time, it may be in part due to an abundance of energy in the meridian that is taking over the cycle at that time.

In addition to the major twelve meridians, there are also eight extraordinary meridians. Of the eight, only two are widely utilized: the central meridian and the governing meridian. These two meridians run up the front and back of the midline respectively and act as guardians of the body and regulators of the major twelve meridians.

Central and Governing Meridians

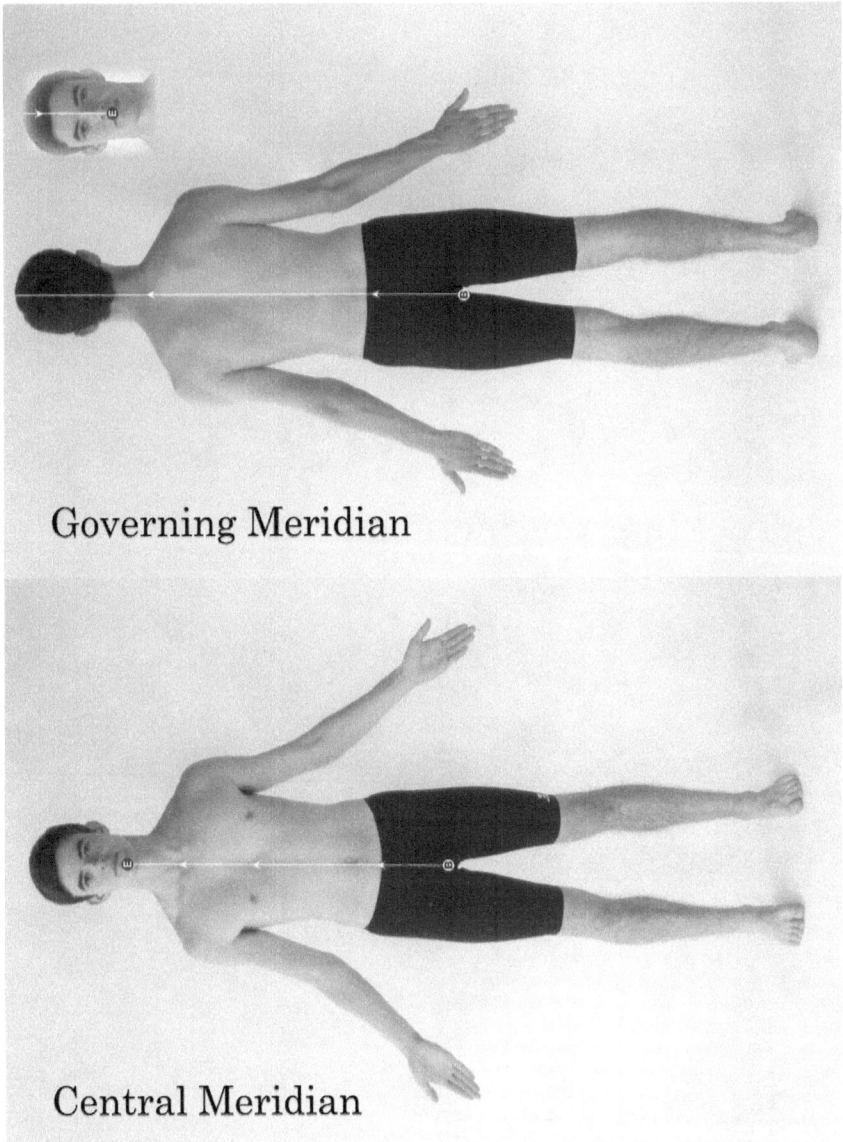

Figure 3: Central and Governing Meridians

Fire Element Meridians

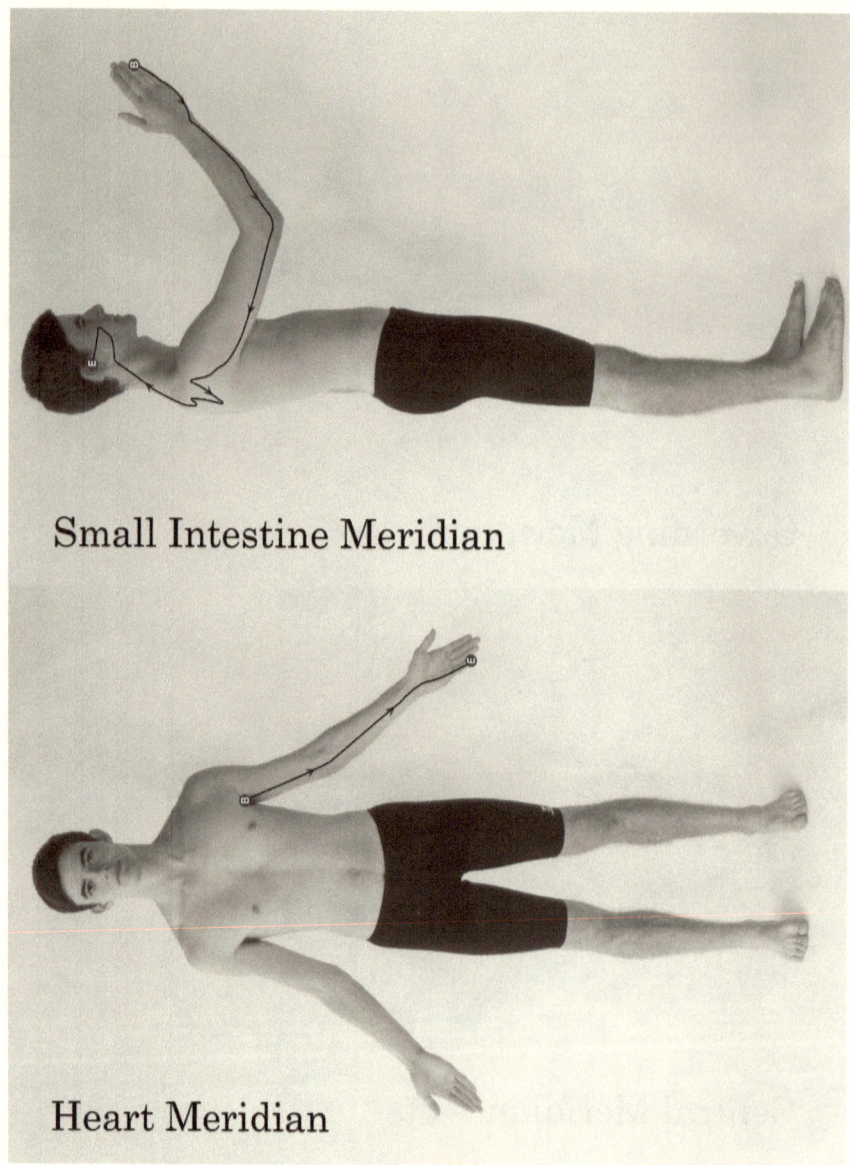

Small Intestine Meridian

Heart Meridian

Figure 4: Heart and Small Intestine Meridians

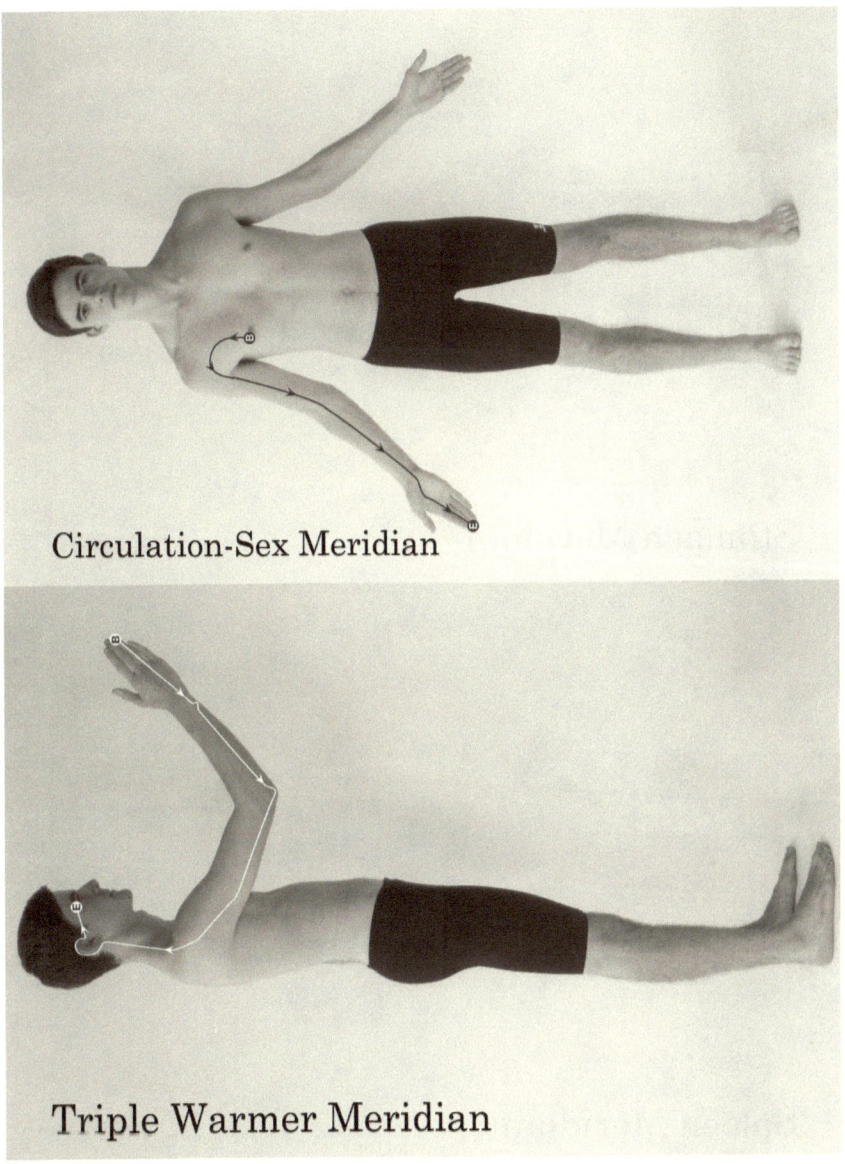

Circulation-Sex Meridian

Triple Warmer Meridian

Figure 5: Triple Warmer and Circulation-Sex Meridians

Earth Element Meridians

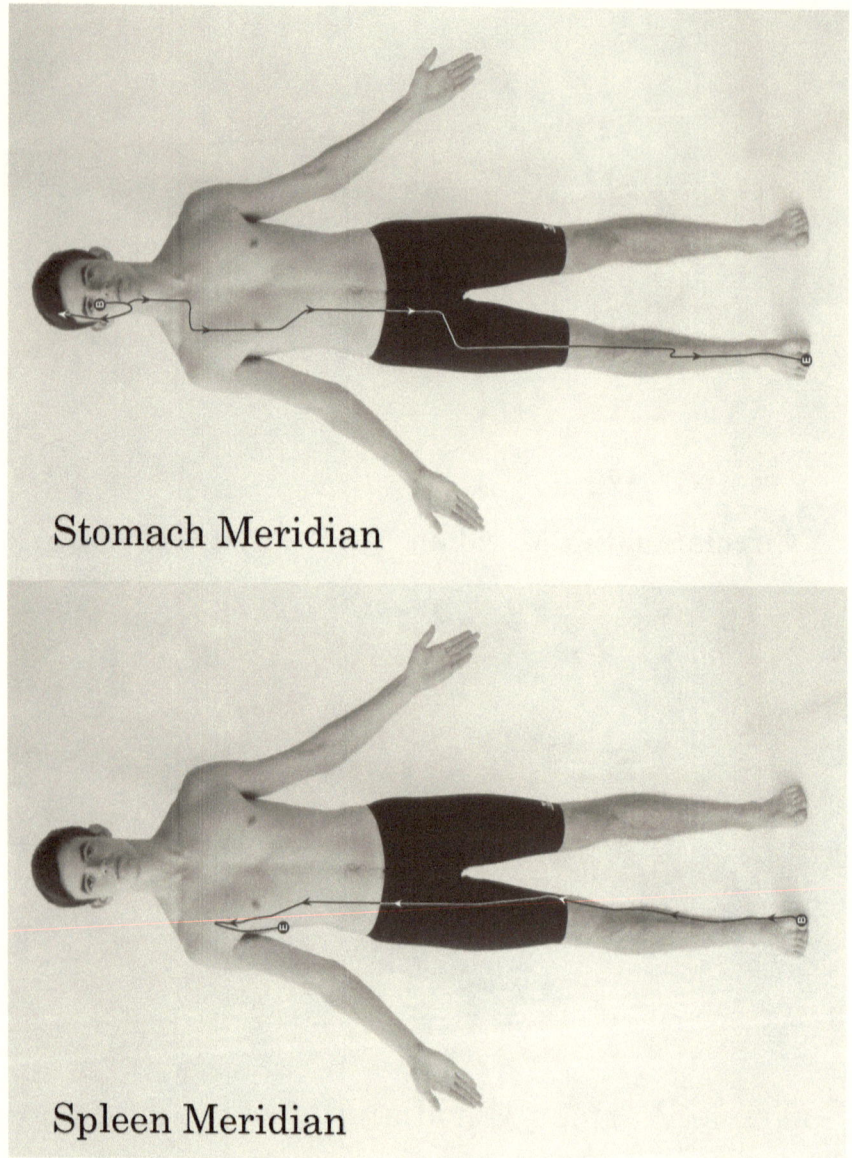

Figure 6: Spleen and Stomach Meridians

Metal Element Meridians

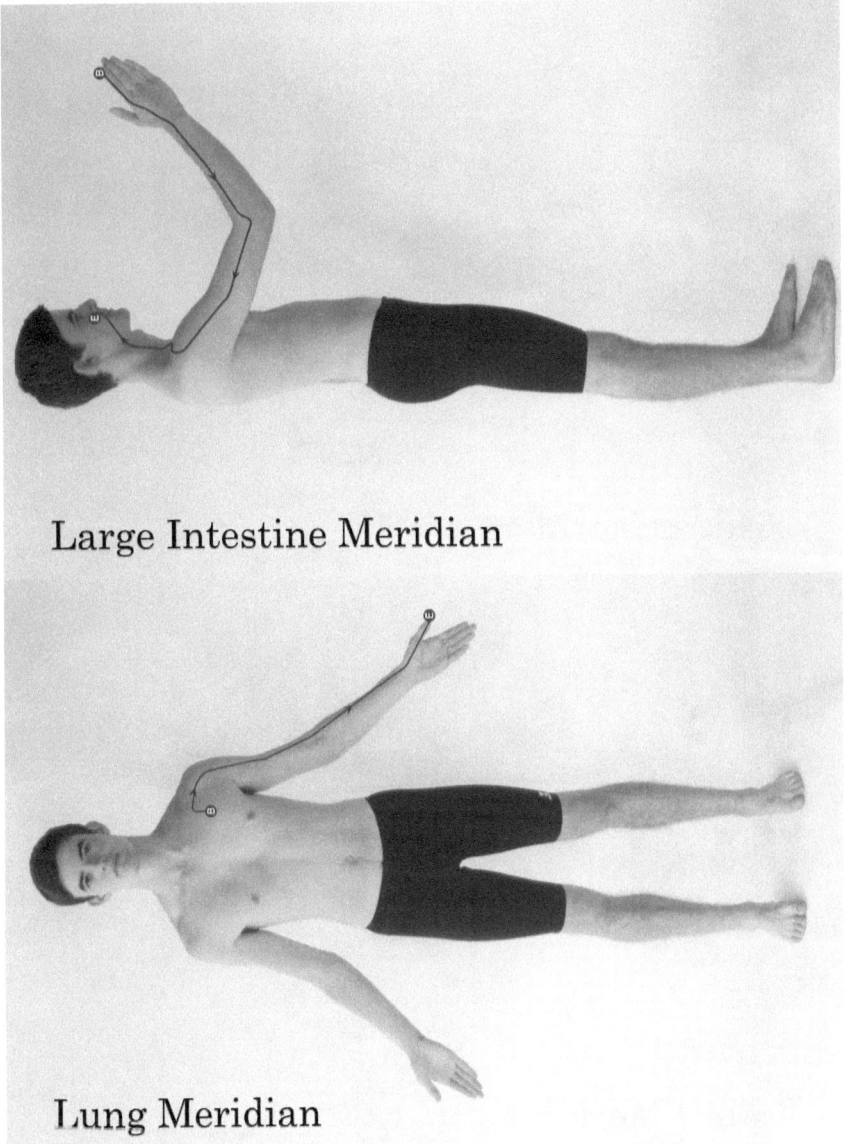

Large Intestine Meridian

Lung Meridian

Figure 7: Lung and Large Intestine Meridians

Water Element Meridians

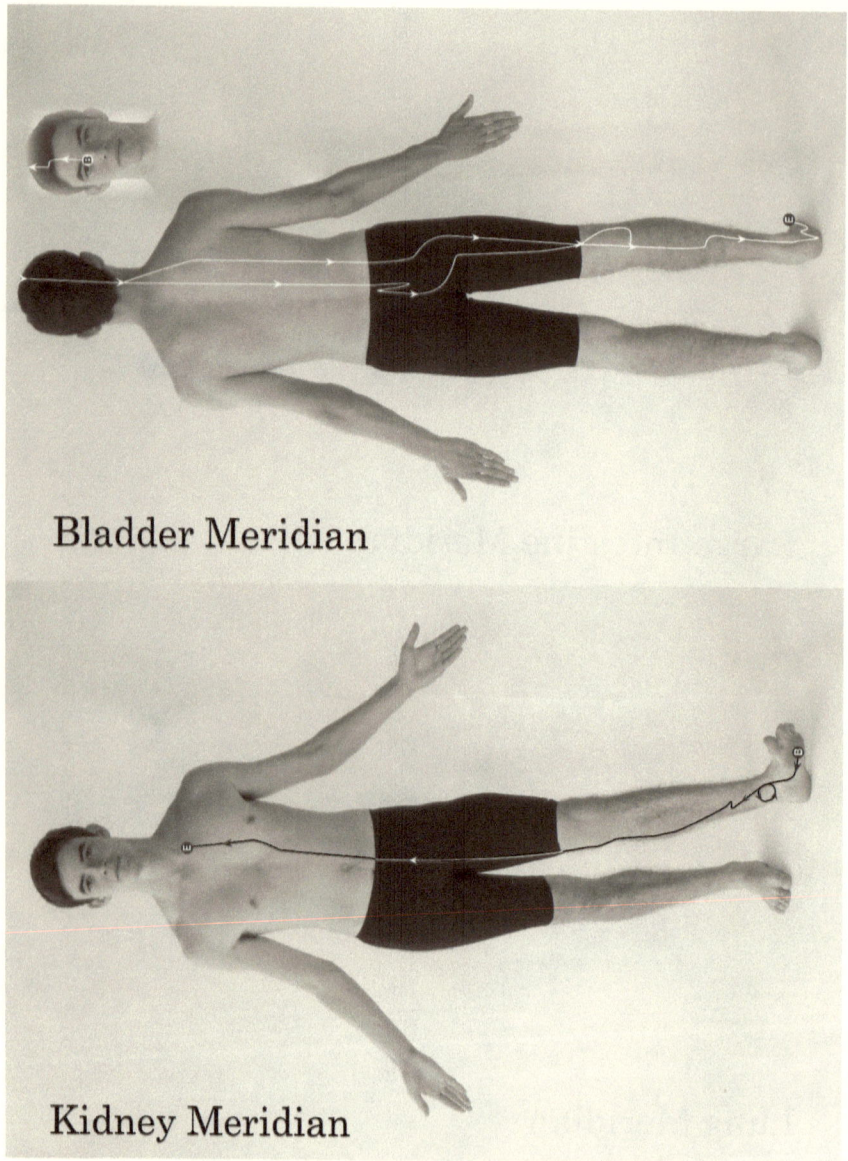

Bladder Meridian

Kidney Meridian

Figure 8: Kidney and Bladder Meridians

Wood Element Meridians

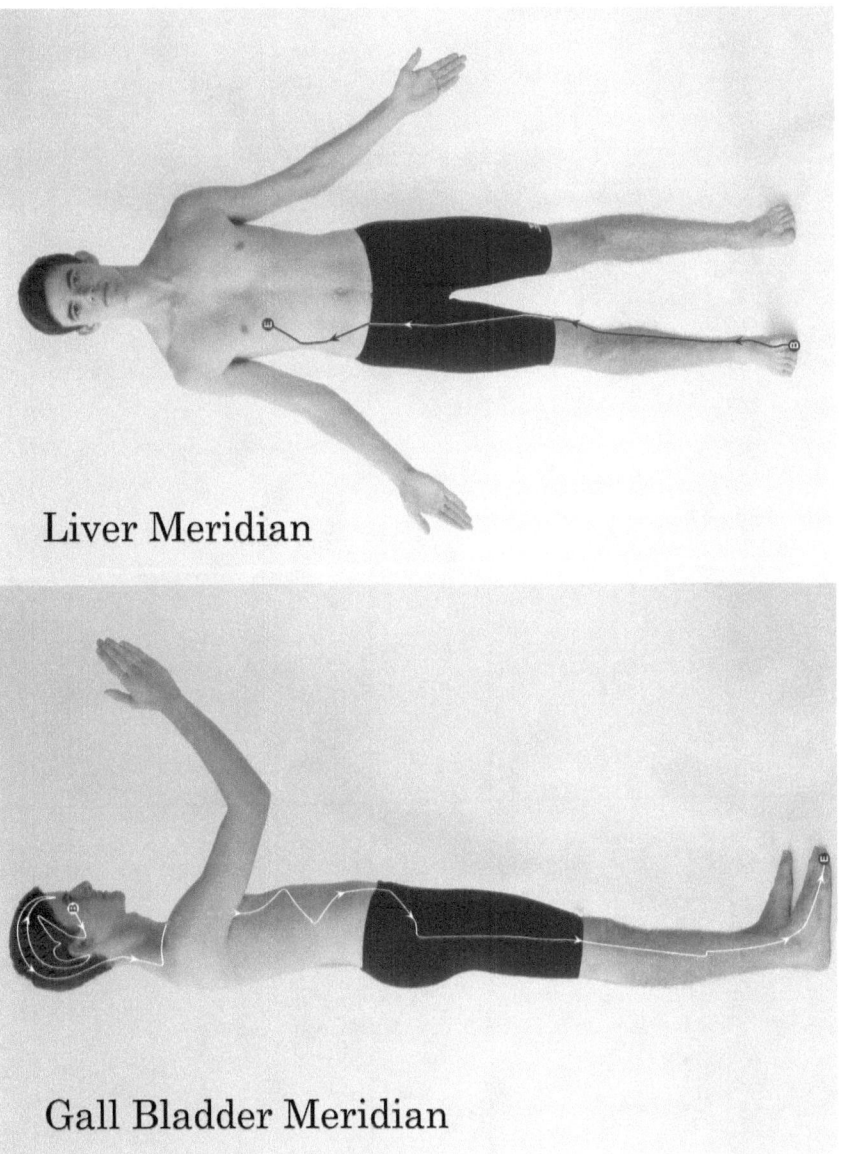

Liver Meridian

Gall Bladder Meridian

Figure 9: Gall Bladder and Liver Meridians

TOOLS

Outstanding additions to your energy evaluation toolkit

Tools for Evaluation

The best way to deliver an effective Reiki session is to first evaluate your client's needs. What issues, if any, is the client dealing with right now? What is the client looking to achieve from this session? Are there chakras or meridians out of balance? Are there any specific areas of energy disturbance? Your client's needs should impact your plan for each session.

In this chapter, we present three evaluation tools: the pendulum, muscle testing, and body scanning. The purpose of these tools is to help you get a clear picture of your client's energy patterns and determine which Reiki protocol will be most beneficial at each session. All three tools can be used for gathering information from the body, and each one has its own merits. The pendulum is primarily used for determining the state of the chakras. Muscle testing is an investigative tool that can help you find not only the priority issue to address, but also the most beneficial Reiki protocol to use to address it. Body scanning is used for pinpointing the exact location of an issue.

When used together, these tools will help you create personalized sessions for your clients that will be most beneficial to their specific needs. Experiment with all three tools and find what works best for you in different situations. Remember everyone is different, and the more tools you have in your toolbox, the more options you have for affecting change.

The Pendulum

A pendulum is an ancient tool used for determining the state of the chakras. It is simple to make and is comprised of a small piece of wood, metal, stone, or other natural material attached at the end of a string or a chain. The practitioner holds the end of the chain and hangs the pendulum over each chakra. Because a chakra is a vortex of energy, it can influence the movement of the pendulum. The direction of movement gives the practitioner information about the health of the chakra. Figure 10 depicts different directions of pendulum movement and their possible interpretations.

Circular movement,
diameter at least 2.5 inches
Clockwise: Chakra is open
Counterclockwise: Open
but is cleaning itself .

Back and forth movement across the body.
Chakra is blocked.
No indication of the type of blockage

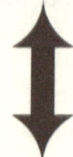

Up and down movement over the body
Chakra is blocked.
Type of blockage:
"I have had enough, don't touch me"

From the right shoulder to the left leg
Chakra is blocked
Type of blockage:
passive emotions

From the left shoulder to the right leg
Chakra is blocked
Type of blockage:
aggressive emotions

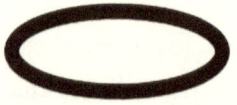

Pendulum moves in the shape of an oval
Chakra is opening up,
but there is still a blockage.
Refere to "blocked" positions
to determine the type.

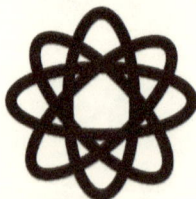

Chaotic movement of the
pendulum indicates
emotional confusion

No movement
Chakra is closed

Figure 10: Pendulum Movements and Possible Interpretations

Using the Pendulum to Evaluate Chakras

1. Start with the client lying face up on the table.
2. Take a deep breath, and clear and calm your mind. This step is very important as it helps you "get out of the way" and stay impartial so you do not influence the movement of the pendulum.
3. Bring the pendulum to the center of the chakra in question.
4. Hold your hand still, and allow the pendulum to move on its own.
5. Record the direction of movement and its interpretation and discuss it with your client. (See Figure 10.)
6. Move to the next chakra and repeat steps 2 to 5.

Using Pendulum to Receive Yes/No Answers

Make the intention as follows:

- Pendulum moves in a line back and forth toward you – "Yes" answer
- Pendulum moves in a line from left to right – "No" answer

To receive the answer:

1. Take a deep breath, and clear and calm your mind. This step is very important as it helps you "get out of the way" and stay impartial so you do not influence the movement of the pendulum.
2. Keep the pendulum in front of you.
3. Formulate a very clear question that can be answered, "Yes" or "No."
4. Keep the pendulum still and allow it to move on its own.
5. Record the answer.

Byosan Reikan-Ho: Focused Healing/Body Scanning

Byosan Reikan-Ho is a fantastic tool for the Reiki practitioner. With this technique, the client's entire body is "scanned" for areas of imbalance, or byosan. This scanning allows the practitioner to hone in on the most beneficial areas of focus, based on the client's issue, in order to have a more productive session.

Byosan Reikan-Ho is an original technique from Master Usui, which can be used either as self-treatment or to help others. The words "Byosan Reikan" describe the energy of an imbalance as detected by the hands. Byosan Reikan literally means energy sensation of sickness (imbalance/ disease). "Byo" means disease or sickness, and "san" means before, ahead, previous, future, or precedence. "Rei" means energy, soul, or spirit, and "kan" means emotion, feeling, or sensation.

A byosan can be present even when the client is unaware of a physical condition. It may show up in a place where it is obvious (over or near an affected or uncomfortable part of the body) or somewhere that seems completely unrelated. An energy blockage or disturbance in one part of the body can affect the energy flow to other parts of the body, so the area where a byosan is found may not always be intuitive based on the issue at hand. By working at the areas found during scanning, you will be balancing a disruptive energy pattern that is making it difficult for the client's natural healing process to be effective.

The ability to sense a byosan will vary greatly from person to person. Some Reiki students will readily detect it, and others will take time to develop this ability. Once attuned to Reiki, your hands become much more sensitive to feeling differences and changes in the body's energies. The more you practice Reiki, the stronger this ability becomes. When detecting a byosan, you will feel sensations, such as tingling, tickling, pulsating, piercing, buzzing, pain, numbness, heat, or cold. These sensations are called hibikis. When areas of extreme disturbances are detected, the hibiki may feel very strong and may travel up your arms. In these cases, it is best to move your hands slightly farther from the body until the sensation is tolerable.

Byosan Reikan-Ho is a great tool to use before the session to evaluate your client or during the session to find and correct imbalances.

Scanning for Byosan

1. Stand or sit near the client and connect to the chi using Reiki.
2. Hold your hands about one to three inches above the body, starting at the head.
3. Slowly move your hands from the top of the client's head to the soles of the feet, passing over all areas of the body. As you move your hands, pay attention to how they feel.
4. When you sense a hibiki, you have found your first byosan and the first area of concentration. At this point, you have two options. You may choose to stop and work on this first area of imbalance until it clears and then move on to find other byosan, or you may choose to scan the entire body noting all areas of imbalance before going back to start working on them. Either method works equally well.

Restoring Balance to the Areas Where Byosan Were Found

1. Place your hands on or close to the body over the affected area.
2. Slowly raise your hands straight above the area until you feel a change in the energy sensation. You may feel a stickiness or magnetism when you reach the appropriate distance from the body.
3. Hold your hands at this height for about five minutes or until you feel a "lightening" of the sensation or intuitively feel that the area is complete.

4. Now continue to raise your hands, stopping at every area of disturbance and clearing it, until you no longer sense the imbalance. Repeat this procedure for each byosan.

Muscle Testing

Muscle testing is a valuable tool for Reiki practitioners. It is a method of biofeedback that can be used to gain insight into the client's current state of health. It involves applying gentle pressure against a muscle's range of motion and observing its behavior. When pressure is applied, the muscle being tested will either "lock" (appear strong and hold in place) or "unlock" (appear weak or soft). These responses in the muscle give the tester information about the energy flow in the body and how the body responds to different stimuli. Muscle testing is a valuable tool for Reiki practitioners to learn, because it can provide very useful information. Many of the Reiki protocols taught in this book benefit from or rely on the use of muscle testing.

This chapter teaches a method of muscle testing which uses one muscle as an indicator for the body as a whole. This method is based on the teachings of Touch for Health, a system of kinesiology created by Dr. John Thie. Touch for Health is a comprehensive system of natural health care that uses muscle testing and simple reflexes to balance the body's energies to promote health, vitality, and wellness. [2] Training in Touch for Health is available all over the world for laypeople and professionals alike. [3]

---

[2] John Thie, DC, and Matthew Thie, M. Ed. *Touch for Health: The Complete Edition.* DeVorss & Company, 2005.

[3] While Touch for Health training is not required for the techniques in this book, those with the training will have more options to go further with the techniques and give the client more tangible feedback.

Since the goal of muscle testing is to get helpful feedback from the body, it is important to make sure that the body is in a state where it can supply accurate answers before you begin the testing. This first involves making sure that the muscle being tested can both lock and unlock. For the techniques in this book, we will use the brachioradialis muscle in the arm as our indicator muscle. Brachioradialis runs between the upper and lower arm and works to bend the elbow and turn the wrist. It is easily tested with the client lying on a table which is why we will be using it here.

Testing the Brachioradialis Muscle

1. Have the client lie face up on the table.
2. With elbows resting on the table and thumbs facing up, have the client bend one arm at the elbow to slightly more than ninety degrees.
3. Apply gentle, steady pressure for about two seconds to the forearm as if to extend the elbow and bring the arm back to the table. The arm should lock and hold firm against your gentle pressure. Test both arms. (See figure 11.)
4. If one or both arms do not hold firm or lock, then the energy flow must be adjusted before continuing.
   a. If both arms felt soft, or unlocked, gently rub up and down on the client's spine over T12 for a few seconds, then retest the muscles. (See figure 12.)
   b. If only one unlocked, rub firmly between the fifth and sixth ribs on the front left side of the client's body and on either side of the spine between T5 and T6. (See figure 12.) Then hold the hand lightly across the forehead. Do these exercises for about ten to twenty seconds. Test both arms again, and the muscles should now lock.[4]

---

[4]   John Thie, DC, and Matthew Thie, M. Ed. *Touch for Health: The Complete Edition*. DeVorss & Company, 2005. 116–117.

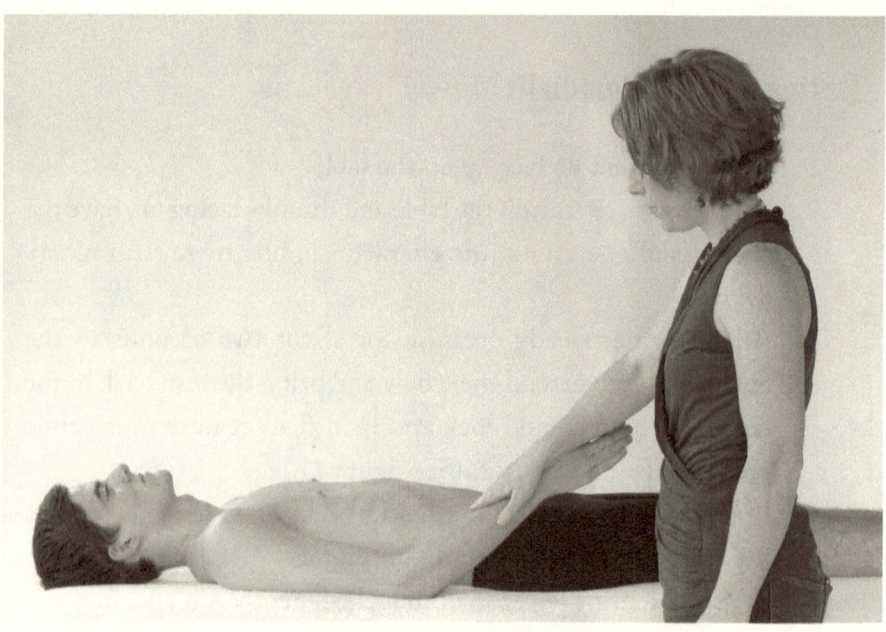

Figure 11: Testing the Brachioradialis Muscle

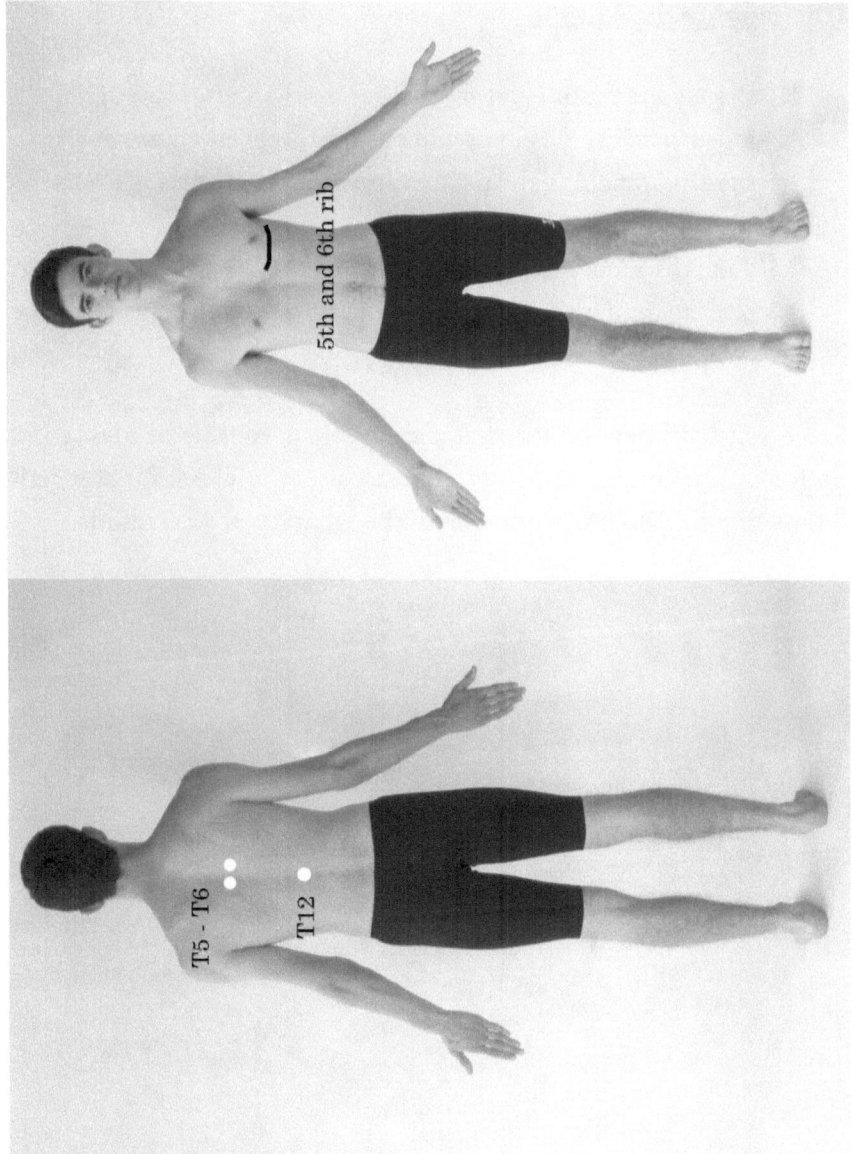

Figure 12: T5, T6, T12, and 5th and 6th Rib Position

Once you have a muscle that will lock, you must make sure that it can also unlock. The following is the procedure for challenging the muscle to ensure it will give both lock and unlock responses.

<u>Challenging the Muscle</u>

1. Place your thumb and first finger on the muscular part of the forearm below the elbow and push them together lengthwise on the arm, pinching the muscle. Immediately retest the muscle. It should unlock. (See figure 13.)
2. Take the same position with the fingers as above, but this time, push apart on the muscle. Immediately retest. The muscle should now lock. (See figure 14.)

Once you have determined that the muscle is capable of giving you both lock and unlock responses, you can use it to check for energetic scrambling that might interfere with the accuracy of your results.

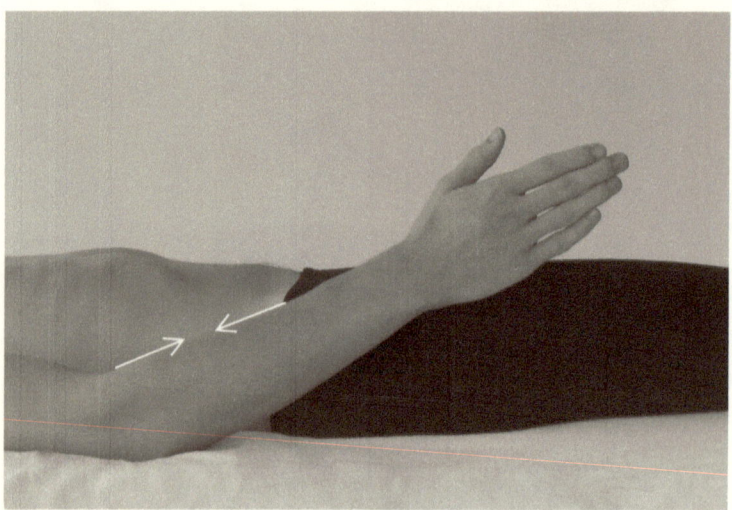

Figure 13: Unlocking the Muscle

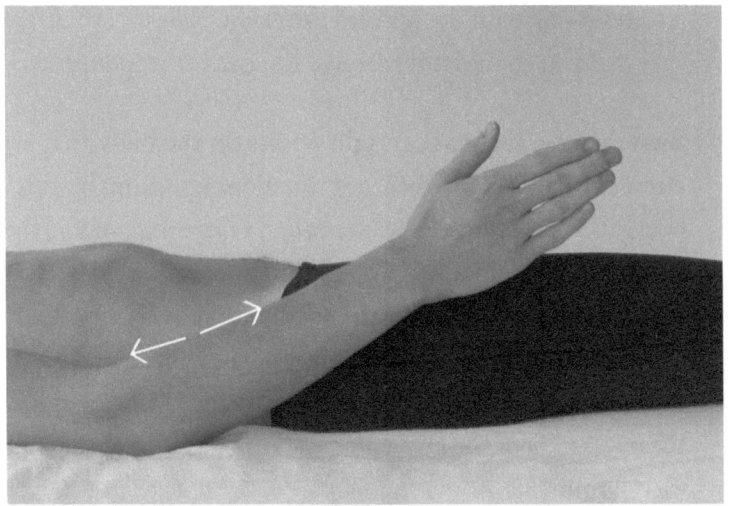

Figure 14: Locking the Muscle

Checking for Energetic Scrambling

Perform the following tests:

- **Central Meridian** - This meridian runs up the front of the body and can have a great effect on muscle testing results as well as on focus and concentration.

  1. Run a hand up the front of the body from the pubic bone to the bottom lip, staying within three inches of the body. Immediately test the indicator muscle. It should lock.
  2. Now run the hand down the front of the body in the same manner and immediately test the muscle again. It should unlock. End by running the hand up the front of the body again.
  3. If you get opposite results (i.e., the muscle stays locked when the meridian is run downward and unlocks when the meridian is run upward), flush the meridian by running a hand up and down the front of the body several times,

finishing with the upward direction. Retest both directions, and you should now receive the correct responses.

- **Switching** - There are certain points on the body that act like circuit breakers and when not functioning optimally can cause energetic confusion. These are called switching points. The first includes the endpoints of the kidney meridian, located in the two soft spots just below the medial points of the collarbone. The second includes the endpoints of the central and governing meridians, located above and below the lips. The third includes the beginning of the governing meridian located at the tailbone. (See figure 15.)

  1. Test each set of points by having the client touch each point in the set as you test the indicator muscle. The muscle should lock.
  2. If any of the points unlock the indicator muscle, rub firmly on each point for a few seconds.
  3. Touch these points again and retest the muscle. It should now lock.

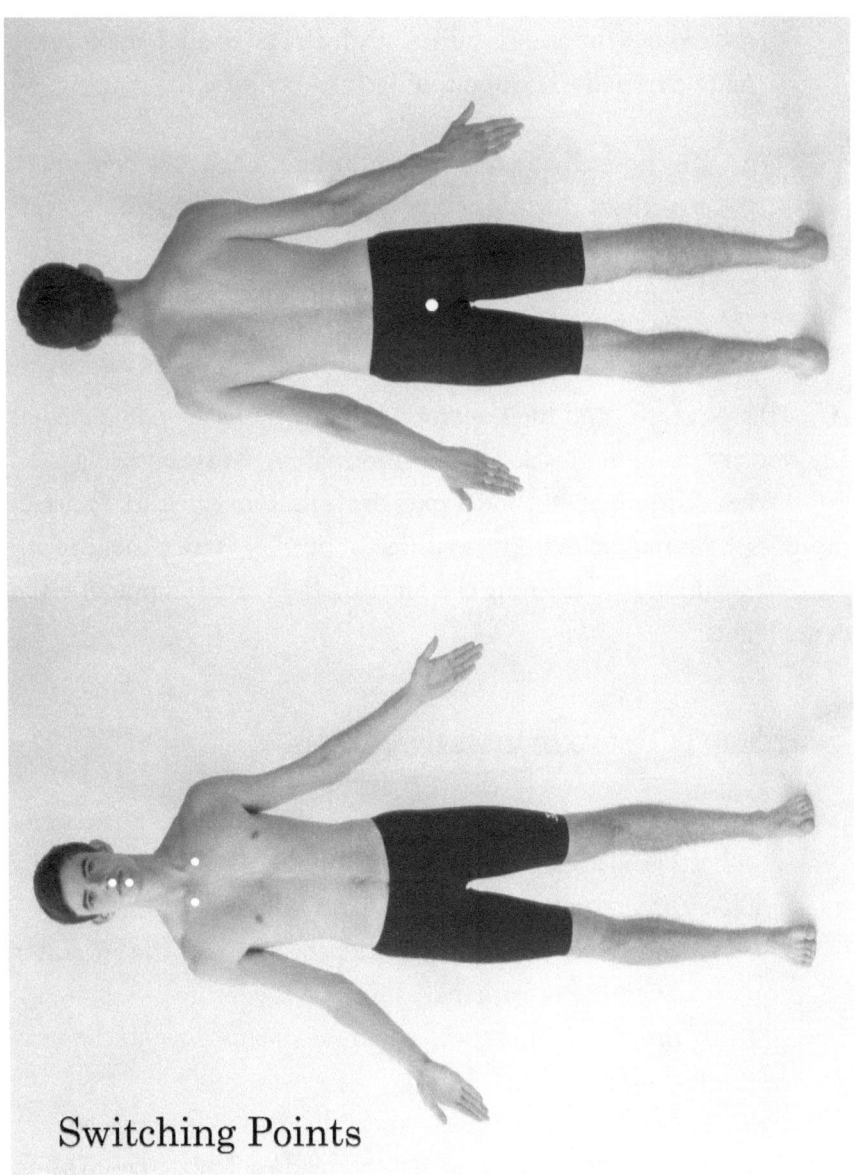

Switching Points

Figure 15: Switching Points

- **Hydration** – Our bodies are largely made of water, and we need it to survive. Without proper hydration, none of our body systems function optimally, including our energy system. This test ensures the body is sufficiently hydrated to allow appropriate muscle responses during testing.

  1. To test for hydration, tug on the hair at the back of the neck to activate the skin and test the indicator muscle at the same time. The muscle should lock.
  2. If the muscle does not lock, have the client drink some filtered water, and then retest the muscle. It should now lock.[5]

After these pretests and their appropriate corrections are completed, if any, you are ready to muscle test for information. Muscle testing is an art. It takes a certain finesse and a good deal of practice to learn to detect the changes in muscle response in different people. Have patience with yourself while you are learning the process. The more you practice, the easier it gets!

Using Muscle Testing to Evaluate Chakras

1. Follow the procedure above to use brachioradialis as an accurate indicator muscle.
2. Check and correct for energetic scrambling.
3. Place one hand over the root chakra and test the indicator muscle with the other hand.
   a. If the muscle locks, the chakra is open. Move to the next chakra.
   b. If the muscle unlocks, keep the hand over the chakra and test the muscle while you read each statement in the

---

[5] John Thie, DC, and Matthew Thie, M. Ed. *Touch for Health: The Complete Edition*. DeVorss & Company, 2005. 36–46.

"Possible Chakra Imbalances" list below. The muscle will unlock when you find the priority reason for the imbalance.

4.   Repeat this procedure for each chakra.

Possible Chakra Imbalances

- Chakra is blocked and overstimulated.
- Chakra is blocked with aggressive emotions.
- Chakra is blocked with passive emotions.
- Chakra has a general blockage.
- Chakra is cleaning itself.
- Chakra is partially blocked.
- Emotional confusion.
- Chakra is closed.

DESIGNING AN INDIVIDUALIZED SESSION

Suggestions for getting the most out of your Reiki sessions

Making It Personal

In the next few chapters, you will learn a great many protocols for working with energy as part of a Reiki session. Every Reiki session is unique and should be built around the needs of the client. The protocols chosen must be those that will work best for the client at that particular time. By using the evaluation tools taught earlier in this book, you will be able to hone in on what is most needed by your client and design a session that is both beneficial and efficient.

Keeping a Log

It is useful and validating to both you and your client to be able to see the progress resulting from your sessions. Therefore, it is essential to get a picture of the client's starting point through verbal dialogue and energy evaluations, and to keep logs of each session. Over time, these records will provide insight into the client's energy patterns (i.e., unstable chakras, imbalanced meridians, the dynamic between the emotional state and blockage movement, and more).

The list below is a starting point and can be expanded as necessary. Any information that you feel would be helpful in caring for your client should be kept in the log.

<u>At a minimum, the log should include the following:</u>

- the date
- any significant information your client gives you (emotional or physical traumas, illnesses, current issues, etc.)
- the results of your initial evaluation (e.g., chakra patterns, meridian imbalances, other energetic disturbances, postural evaluations, and visual observations)

- protocols and other healing tools that you chose for the session (e.g., essential oils, crystals, meditations, and healing music)
- any results of the session (significant comments or changes the client has at the conclusion of the session)

Planning the Session

Below, you will find our approach for how to lay out a session using the protocols you will learn in this book. Any other protocols or techniques that you have in your personal toolkit can be added to this procedure. The idea is to really listen, and do an evaluation that gives you a clear picture of your client's current energy profile and future goals. From there, you will work to find exactly what protocols or techniques will be the most helpful at the time of the balance.

Instructions

1. Evaluation:
   a. First talk with your client. Are there any issues that the client is currently dealing with that are causing stress? Is there any pain? Is there anything in particular that the client would like to focus on during the session? Make note of your client's responses in your log.
   b. Perform a preliminary evaluation. Make note of postural issues, visual observations, energetic disturbances, the client's emotional state, etc.
   c. Use one or more of the following methods to evaluate chakras, meridians, or other energy disturbances, based on your needs, and note the findings in your log. (See the "Tools" chapter for more information.)
      i. Pendulum
      ii. Muscle Testing
      iii. Byosan Reikan-Ho

2. Find the Balancing Methods.

    a. Look at the chart in figure 16. All the protocols taught in this book are listed under four categories, mental and emotional protocols, acute protocols, standard protocols and closing protocols. (All protocol categories may not be required for every session.) Use either muscle testing or the pendulum to find the protocols to be used for this session and the order in which to perform them. Start by finding the first category of protocols. Test each category until you have a change in response from your chosen tool. Next test each protocol in that category for a change in response. This is your first protocol. Record the result in your log.

    b. Test through the categories again as in the previous step, looking for the next category of protocol to use. It may be the same category or a new one. Again test through each protocol for an indicator change. This will be the second protocol you perform. Record the result in your log. Continue this procedure until there is no longer a change in response from your tool when you test through the categories.

3. Perform the required protocols in the order determined in step 2.
4. Ask your client for feedback on the session. Record any comments in your log.

Mental and Emotional Protocols	Stress Release	Emotional Release	Past Life Regression	
Acute Protocols	Chakra Shooting	Chakra Spreading	Tapping	Pulsing
Standard Protocols	Basic Hand Positions / Reiki Meridian	Alternative Hand Positions / Reiki Spiral	Byosan Reikan-Ho	Reiji
		Balancing Chakras w/ Marmas		
Closing Protocols	Basic Ayurvedic	Spirit Mind Balance	Chakra Emotional Balance	Zenshin Koketsu Ho / Ketsueki Koukan Ho

Figure 16: Reiki Protocols Chart

MENTAL AND EMOTIONAL PROTOCOLS

Methods for relieving mental and emotional stress and trauma

Emotions and Our Health

Emotions are responsible for a high percentage of the issues experienced in our bodies, minds, and spirits. When emotions are suppressed, either because they are too painful to experience or because we just don't know how to express them, stress builds up in our bodies and causes things to go out of balance. How can we stop our emotions from causing these imbalances? By learning to allow ourselves to fully experience these emotions and release the stressful feelings and issues that are causing us pain and holding us back.

Emotional protocols are an important part of every Reiki treatment. They help the body to release blockages that are being held by stuck emotions. Very often, physical pain and other seemingly unrelated issues are relieved by addressing the emotions.

Important: Emotional release and past life regression should not be used in the same session. Using more than one of these protocols at a time could release a considerable amount of imbalanced energy too quickly. This might leave your client unprepared for the sudden changes and might delay the recovery or cause discomfort. Always follow this rule: slow is good. Gradual changes give your clients time to adjust energetically, emotionally, and spiritually. Gradual changes lead to permanent changes.

Stress Release

One of the most powerful protocols for emotional release is incredibly simple. Place your hand on your forehead and think about the problem. That's all there is to it! Think about it. What do you do when life throws you a curve ball? Most people put their hand on their forehead and say, "Oh no, what am I going to do?" This is a natural response to the stress being experienced.

The bumps on the forehead above the eyebrows are the key to this and many other protocols for emotional healing. In traditional Chinese medicine, these points are called "Seat of the Soul." In Ayurveda, they are called Bhruh Madhya. In kinesiology, they are called the frontal eminences, neurovascular points that, when touched lightly, encourage blood flow to the area. This increased blood flow helps bring focus from the back brain, the fight-or-flight center, to the forebrain, the logical thinking center. This in turn helps us see the issue at hand more clearly, release the stressful emotions associated with it, and think through it toward a logical solution.[6]

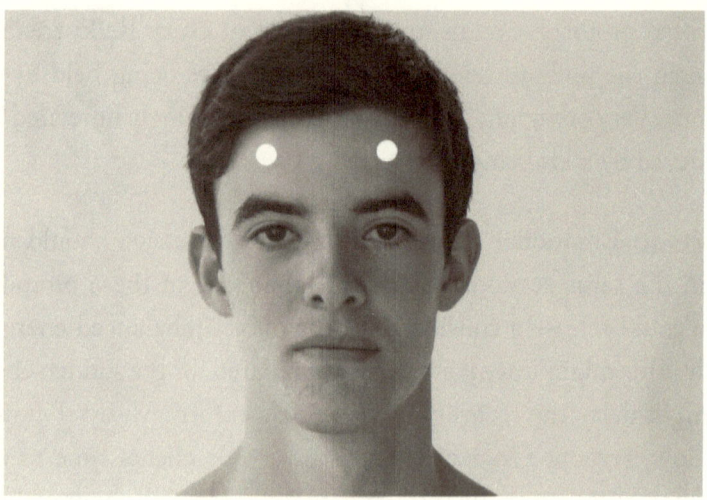

Figure 17: Emotional Points

This protocol can be used anytime, anywhere for instant help with emotional overload.

Instructions

1. Identify the stressful issue.
2. Have the client put a hand across the forehead.

---

[6] John Thie, DC, and Matthew Thie, M. Ed. *Touch for Health: The Complete Edition*. DeVorss & Company, 2005. 38–40.

3. Ask the client to think or talk through the issue in as much sensory detail as possible (i.e., see it, hear it, feel it, smell it, and taste it).

4. Hold this position until one of you yawns or sighs or the client feels relief and feels ready to stop. (Often a yawn or sigh from the client or practitioner is an indication that an energy shift has occurred and the correction is complete.)

Emotional Release

This protocol is done by "unlocking" the emotional points on the forehead, just above the center of the eyebrows. These are the same points used in the previous stress release protocol.

The beauty of this protocol is that the client does not have to re-experience the emotions. The client might not know about these particular repressed emotions because of a state of denial or other blocking mechanism. When strong, shocking, negative emotions are experienced, they can end up stored in any part of the body in the form of imbalanced energy. This creates a blockage, which can lead to physical issues or disease.

The images in our memories are attached to emotions. When we bring up a picture in our mind, we are filled with feelings that accompany that memory or thought image. A stressful memory or thought is associated with negative emotions, such as fear or anger. The goal of emotional release is to find these stressful images and release them with all their attached negative emotions.

Instructions

1. Position yourself at the head of the table.
2. Put both hands on the top of the client's head.

3. With one hand draw the power symbol, emotional symbol, and power symbol again over the top of the client's head. (Refer to your second degree Reiki manual for these symbols.)

4. Gently draw a counterclockwise circle over the right emotional point nine times.

5. Repeat for the left point. You have now "unlocked" the emotional gate.

6. Keep the tips of your fingers on the points.

7. Encourage the client to relax and go into a deep meditative state. (See the appendix for an example of a simple meditation that can be used for this purpose.)

8. Once the client is relaxed, ask the following question: "Do you see any color or image associated with negative emotions?"

9. After receiving the answer, ask the client to repeat after you the following affirmation: "I willingly and lovingly release [insert the name of the image from the previous step] and all negative emotions associated with it and fill myself with unconditional love and light."

10. You will feel the flow of energy as the emotion is being released. Keep the tips of your fingers on the points until you feel the energy flow has subsided.

11. Gently draw a clockwise circle over the right point five times.

12. Repeat for the left point. You have now "put a separator" between emotions.

13. Repeat steps 4 to 12 two more times with one difference: the last time through, for steps 11 and 12, do nine clockwise circles to "lock" the points instead of five clockwise circles.

14. Follow this protocol with one of the standard protocols presented later in this book.

Important: Do not repeat steps 4 to 12 if you feel that your hands are getting too hot. It might indicate that the repressed emotion that has just been released is very powerful, and the client may need time to adjust. Finish the release that is already underway and lock the emotional points by gently drawing nine clockwise circles over both the right and left points nine times.

Past Life Regression

Everything that is in our minds is real to us and affects our responses to life's events and our interactions with other people. Blockages in our energy can impede us from moving forward and achieving our goals. Past life regression is said to release blockages that were acquired in previous lives so our life lessons may be seen more clearly. The concept of reincarnation is an organic part of many belief systems and may or may not be part of your client's beliefs. Some practitioners utilize this technique metaphorically, or describe the experiences as possibly ancestral, being passed down through the family tree. Regardless of how you view past life regression, or whatever your beliefs are about it, the technique is very helpful in balancing stuck emotions and unconscious blockages that may be impeding the realization of full potential.

You as a practitioner will not be able to see what your client sees, but you will be able to get a sense of the emotions in your hands. Pay attention. When your client goes through a very painful experience, it is your job to help by asking the client to step out and observe the situation from a distance or to just end the regression.

Instructions

1. Position yourself at the head of the table.
2. Put both hands on the top of the client's head.
3. With one hand, draw the power symbol, the emotional symbol, and the power symbol again over the top of the client's head. (Refer to your second degree Reiki manual for these symbols.)

4. Put the client into a deep meditative state using the meditation below. Say each of the statements in a soothing voice, pausing a few seconds between each one.

a. Sink into the table.

b. Relax your feet, legs, and so on, continuing up your body until you reach the top of your head.

c. Imagine yourself rising slightly above your body, just a few inches. Feel that it is safe and you can come back any time you want. Now go back to your body.

d. Rise over your body again, higher this time. Now go back to your body again.

e. Rise over your body again. Go up through the ceiling of this room, through _____ (mention other floors, if any), through the roof of this building.

f. Fly into the sky.

g. In the distance, you see a very tall mountain.

h. Fly toward this mountain, and land on the top.

i. The mountain is beautiful. It is covered with a peaceful garden with a small pond in the center.

j. You are greeted by your guardian angel.

k. Your guardian angel takes you by the hand and leads you toward the border of the garden.

l. There are bridges that go into the white clouds that surround the mountain.

m. Each bridge represents a passage to one of your past lives.

n. Choose one of the bridges and start crossing.

o. Your guardian angel comes with you and invisibly escorts you in your past life to protect you from harm.

p. You are walking into the cloud, and when you emerge on the other side of the bridge, you are in one of your past lives.

5. Ask the following questions to help guide the client in the process:
   a. Are you a boy or a girl?
   b. How old are you?
   c. What is your name?
   d. Where are you?
   e. Do you feel safe?
   f. Do you have any family or friends?

6. After you help to establish the identity, ask, "Would you like to explore more?"
7. Continue the dialogue by asking questions based on what the client tells you.
8. When nothing significant happens, ask, "Would you like to move forward to the next important event in your life?"
9. If the answer is "No," continue to ask questions about what is going on.
10. If the answer is "Yes," say, "Let's move forward to the next important event in your life."
11. Ask the following questions:
    a. How old are you?
    b. Where are you?
    c. Do you have a family?
    d. And any other question that might be appropriate based on what you learned before about this life.

12. Repeat steps 6 to 11 until you reach the end of the life.
13. At the end of the life, continue with the following "closing" meditation:
    a. Let's move forward into the light.
    b. Do you see anyone? Is there anyone greeting you? (There might be family members or deities.)
       i. If the answer is "Yes," ask if there is a message or conversation or a last good-bye and let the client experience the light a little more (ten to twenty seconds).

> Do not let the client linger too long in this state. It is pleasant, but there is no practical reason to stay in it.
>
> ii. If the answer is "No," ask the client to go back to the bridge.

c. Let's walk back over the bridge, through the cloud, back to the garden on the top of the mountain.

d. You are greeted by your guardian angel.

e. You both sit near the pond and your guardian angel asks about the lesson you learned during this past life. (Ask the client to talk about this lesson.)

f. Repeat the lesson aloud back to the client.

g. Now let's fly back.

h. Fly back to this building.

i. Go down through the roof, through all the floors.

j. Fly back into this room.

k. Come back into your body, stretch, and end this past life regression.

14. Offer the client a glass of water and press into the point at the center of the ball of the foot where there is a little indentation. This is the first point on the kidney meridian, and it helps to ground the client.

15. Talk to the client about the important points of this past life.

16. Follow the past life regression with a standard protocol, such as the alternative hand positions.

ACUTE PROTOCOLS

Chakra balancing for acute stress and trauma, and
some specific methods for moving energy

Chakra Balancing Protocols for
Acute Stress and Trauma

At times of severe stress and trauma, the chakras may have a difficult time accepting healing. It is at these times that it may be necessary to "prep" the chakras to receive energy. Without first addressing the chakras in this manner, it may be difficult to get to the underlying issues and promote healing. The chakra protocols in this chapter are not meant to be used on their own. They should always be followed by a standard protocol, as part of a complete Reiki session. These protocols should also be used sparingly, and only in situations where the client is in distress. For best results, perform the chosen protocol, follow with either the basic or alternative hand positions, (presented in the next chapter, "Standard Protocols"), and then end the session with one of the closing protocols described later in this book.

Important: As a general rule, chakra shooting, chakra spreading, emotional release and past life regression should not be used in the same session. (See previous chapter.) Using more than one of these protocols at a time could release a considerable amount of imbalanced energy too quickly. This might leave your client unprepared for the sudden changes and might delay the recovery or cause discomfort. Always follow this rule: slow is good. Gradual changes give your clients time to adjust energetically, emotionally, and spiritually. Gradual changes lead to permanent changes.

Chakra Shooting

Chakra shooting is a simple protocol that helps to add additional energy to closed chakras. It is used when most of the chakras are closed as a result of prolonged and continued stress.

Instructions

1. Have the client stand while holding onto a chair or table for support. (This is to ensure the client does not fall forward or backwards while you are working.)
2. Stand at the client's right side, so you can easily reach both the front and back of the body.
3. Using the sequence below, hold your hands four to five inches from the body, and send chi in each position until the flow stops. Once the energy has subsided, move on to the next location.
   a. Place your right hand over the root chakra (in front of the body) and your left hand over the crown chakra.
   b. Place both of your hands over the sacral chakra (front and back).
   c. Place both of your hands over the solar plexus chakra (front and back).
   d. Place both of your hands over the heart chakra (front and back).
   e. Place both of your hands over the throat chakra (front and back).
   f. Place both of your hands over the third eye chakra (front and back).

4. To finish, swipe three times down the energy field, both in front and in back of the client's body, from the crown chakra to the feet. Take care not to touch the body.
5. Follow this protocol with a main session protocol.

Chakra Spreading

Chakra spreading is used after a major traumatic event, such as the death of a friend or family member, an accident, major surgery, divorce, or any other life-altering event. It should be done as soon as possible after the traumatic event to minimize the impact of imbalanced energy. Always do this protocol at the beginning of the session.

Instructions

1. Start with the client lying face up on the table.
2. Begin the session by helping your client relax by using the hand positions on the head or a simple meditation. (See the appendix for a meditation example.)
3. Now move to stand at the client's side to begin the chakra spreading protocol. (During this protocol, your hands should remain in the energy field and should never actually touch the body.)
4. Follow the steps below for each chakra in the following order: crown, third eye, throat, heart, solar plexus, sacral, and root.
   a. Place your hands as high as you can above the chakra. (For the crown chakra, hold your hands about twelve inches from the top of the head.)
   b. Slowly move your hands down toward the body until you feel the energy of the chakra. (The sensation is often described as feeling like putting your hands in warm water.)
   c. As soon as you feel the warmth of the chakra, spread it outward at that height three times with the palms of your hands. If no warmth is detected, start spreading four to five inches above the body.
   d. Move to the next chakra.

5. When you have finished spreading all the chakras, remove the accumulated excess energy by swiping outward from the feet three times.
6. Repeat steps 4 and 5 two more times.
7. Follow this protocol with a main session protocol.

Traditional Japanese Protocols for Moving Energy

Typically, Reiki is performed by holding the hands still over specific areas of the body. This method allows for a steady flow of energy to the client. Sometimes, it is beneficial to create different motions of the hand in order to affect the energy in different ways.

Tapping: Uchi-te Chiyo-ho

Tapping the chi field can relieve stress and tension, improve circulation, and relieve congestion. It can be done as part of a full session or as a standalone approach for specific issues.

Instructions

1. Start at the head and begin tapping or patting the chi field, or the body itself, with your palms or fingertips.
2. Work from the head all the way to the feet and then from the feet all the way back to the head one time.

If using this technique as part of a full session, continue with any other necessary protocols.

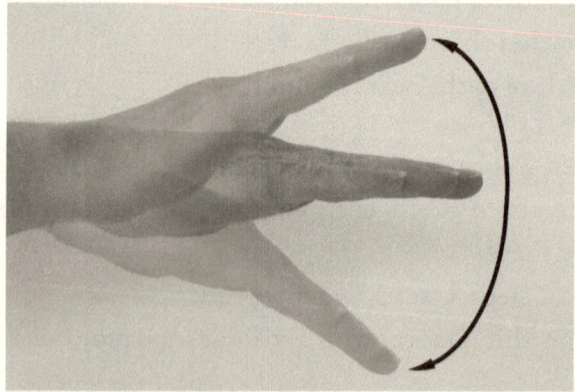

Figure 18: Tapping

Pulsing: Oshi-te Chiryo-ho

Pulsing encourages energy flow and stimulates circulation by drawing energy and awareness to an area of the body. Use this protocol over any area of the body that requires extra energy focus including acupuncture points. Pulsing over specific acupuncture points can stimulate a tingling or warming sensation at the point that radiates along the meridian.

Instructions

1. Hover your hand over the body area needing energy.
2. With the palm facing down, slightly open and close the hand, stretching the fingers of the hand and then relaxing them. The chi emanates from the center of the palm and will take on a pulsing pattern from the action of the hand.

If using this technique as part of a full session, continue with any other necessary protocols.

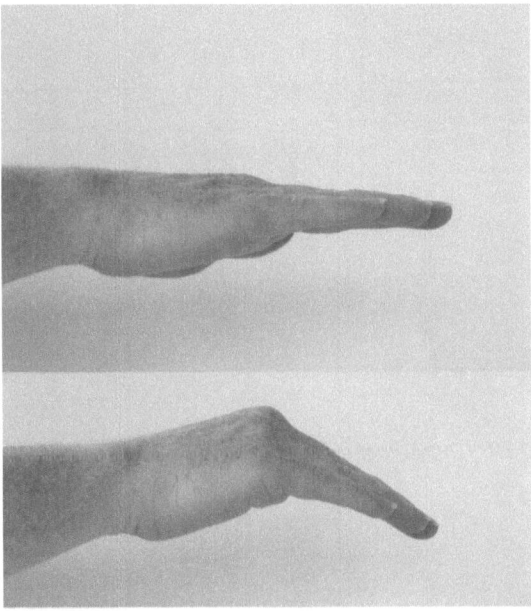

Figure 19: Pulsing

STANDARD PROTOCOLS

Protocols suitable for use as the main Reiki balance

Review of Basic Hand Positions

The basic hand positions are the first way we learn to use Reiki in the West. They give us a procedure to follow and make it easy for beginners and advanced practitioners alike to perform a very beneficial healing session. Each hand position stimulates specific meridians, chakras, marmas, etc. These in turn affect the body and emotions in different ways. By utilizing all the hand positions within a session, all areas of the body receive healing energy and an overall balancing effect is achieved.

Sometimes, it is beneficial to change the order of the hand positions or concentrate on only a few areas, depending on the needs of the client. Figure 20 displays the basic hand positions. The section that follows describes each position and presents some possible benefits of each one. Armed with this knowledge, you will be able to modify a healing session based on your client's needs. For example, if your client is feeling stressed and is suffering from a headache, you may want to spend a little more time on the head and upper chest positions as well as the feet. These areas are related either to neck and shoulder muscles, stress relief, relaxation, headaches, and/or emotional balance.

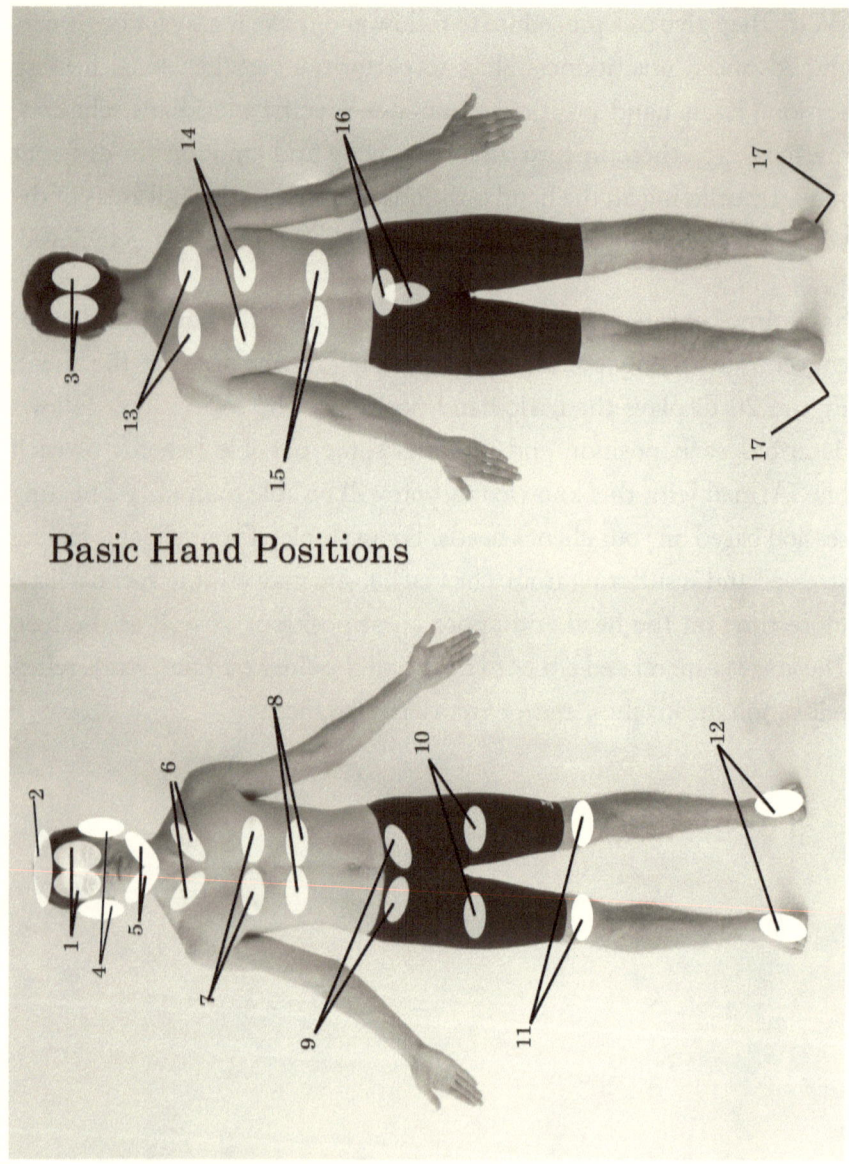

Basic Hand Positions

Figure 20: Basic Hand Positions

The Basic Hand Positions and Their Possible Benefits

Front

1. **Over the Eyes**
    - relieves headaches
    - improves concentration
    - benefits eyes and nose
    - releases suppressed emotions
    - calms the mind
    - balances third eye chakra
    - relaxes back and neck muscles

2. **Over the Head**
    - regulates chi flow
    - balances crown chakra
    - relieves headaches
    - lifts depression
    - relaxes upper legs, hips, and abdominals

3. **Under the Head**
    - reduces stress
    - benefits eyes, lungs, liver, spleen kidney, large intestine, and heart

4. **Over the Ears**
    - calms the mind
    - relieves stress
    - stimulates mental alertness
    - stimulates third eye and heart chakras

5. **Under the Chin**
    - regulates thyroid
    - calms respiratory system
    - relieves neck tension

- clears the mind

6. Over the Chest
- regulates heart function
- calms respiratory system
- balances heart chakra
- maintains immune system
- releases suppressed emotions

7. Over the Heart
- regulates heart rate
- enhances lung function
- balances spleen

8. Over the Solar Plexus
- regulates and enhances digestion
- balances solar plexus chakra
- detoxifies blood
- balances emotions

9. Over the Lower Abdomen
- regulates bladder
- regulates male and female reproductive organs
- stimulates sexual energy
- balances sacral chakra

10. Over the Upper Legs
- regulates blood flow to the legs
- balances root chakra
- relaxes hip flexors

11. Over the Knees
- benefits knees
- balances root chakra

12. Over the Feet

- benefits liver and lungs

Back

13. Over the Upper Back

- stimulates lungs and heart
- calms the mind
- enhances the flow of chi
- releases shoulder tension

14. Over the Middle Back

- benefits liver, gall bladder, and spleen
- enhances the flow of chi

15. Over the Waist

- regulates kidney function
- calms local back pain

16. Over the Tailbone

- benefits kidneys, bladder, and reproductive system
- regulates colon activity
- stimulates chi energy
- balances root chakra
- enhances balance and stability

17. Over the Soles of the Feet

- activates chi
- regulates chi
- maintains equilibrium
- relieves stress
- calms the mind
- provides grounding

Alternative Hand Positions

In 2010, after extensive research into the energy systems, and careful observation, Marina created an alternative sequence of hand positions. This sequence of hand positions was developed out of a desire for faster and more significant results for her clients. Marina found that these new positions were not only highly effective, they were also easier on the client and more comfortable for the practitioner than the basic hand positions. Figure 21 displays the alternative hand positions. The section that follows describes each position and presents some possible benefits of each one. All hand positions are done with the client lying face up.

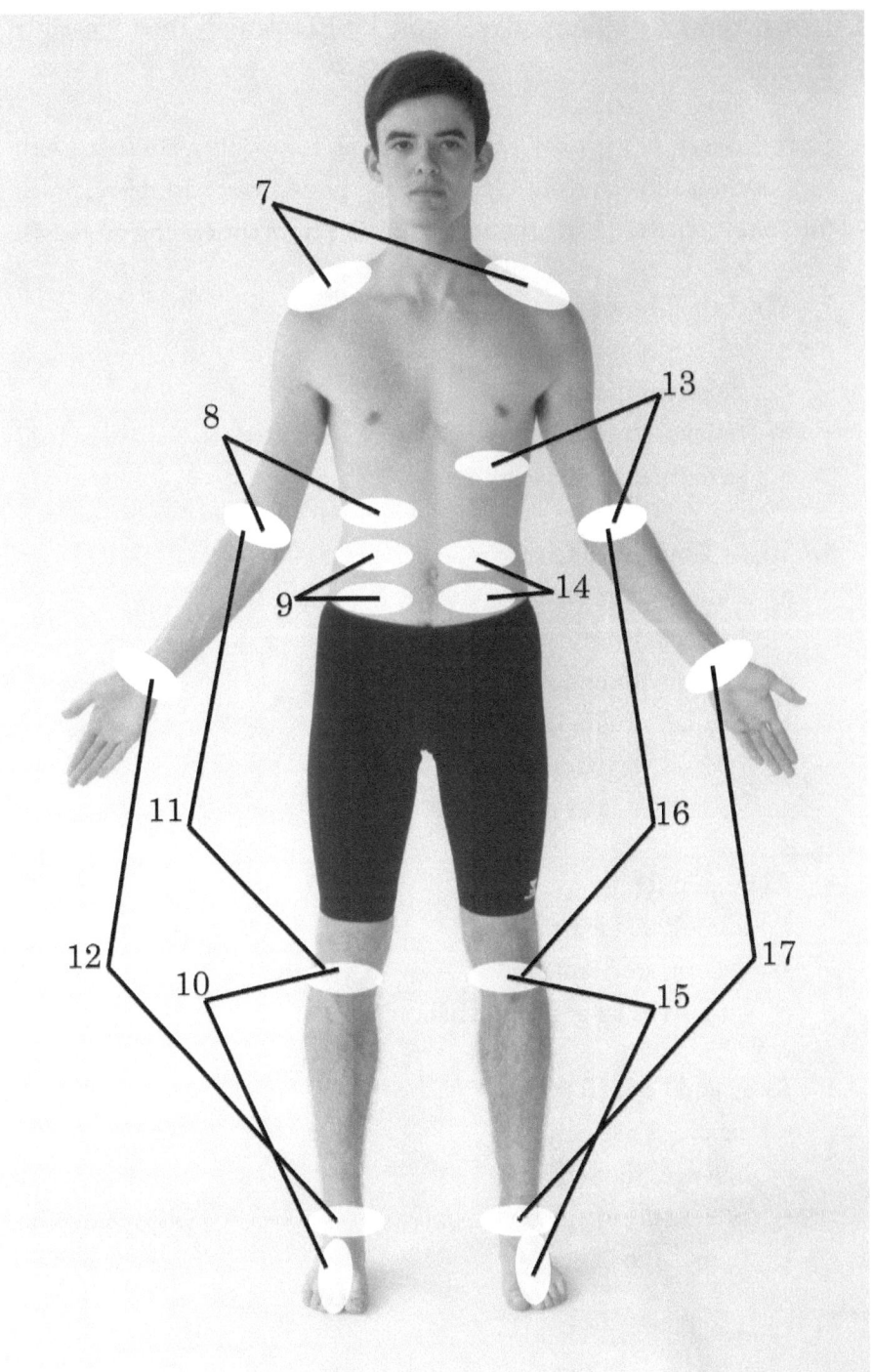

Figure 21: Alternative Hand Positions

Instructions for Alternative Hand Positions and Their Possible Benefits

Start the session with basic hand positions 1 to 6, then continue with the positions shown below. Once all hand positions are complete, finish the session with the basic symmetry balance from the closing protocols.

7. **Over the Shoulder**
   - relieves shoulder pain
   - helps chi flow
   - relieves stress
   - stimulates throat chakra

8. **Right Elbow and Liver**
   - tones bladder
   - balances liver
   - assists with circulation
   - regulates colon function
   - releases stagnant emotions
   - stimulates solar plexus chakra

9. **Abdomen Right**
   - stimulates digestion
   - relieves stagnant chi
   - stimulates solar plexus chakra

10. **Knee and Foot (Right)**
    - relieves knee pain
    - balances root chakra
    - promotes circulation
    - improves balance

11. **Elbow and Knee (Right)**
    - balances root chakra
    - regulates liver

12. Wrist and Ankle (Right)
- balances heart and mind
- balances emotions
- lowers stress
- balances sacral chakra

13. Left Elbow and Spleen
- regulates spleen function
- regulates and detoxifies blood
- strengthens immune system and circulation
- stimulates solar plexus and sacral chakra

14. Abdomen Left
- stimulates digestion
- relieves stagnated chi
- stimulates solar plexus chakra

15. Knee and Foot (Left)
- relieves knee pain
- balances root chakra
- promotes circulation
- improves balance

16. Elbow and Knee (Left)
- balances root chakra
- regulates spleen

17. Wrist and Ankle (Left)
- balances heart and mind
- balances emotions
- lowers stress
- balances sacral chakra

Intuitive Healing: Reiji

Intuition is a natural part of our sense system. It is our ability to read and understand other people's energy bodies and the flow of chi in the environment. Everyone has it, but not everyone is listening. For thousands of years, martial artists and healers have used intuition to assess the environment for danger, to find imbalances that cause disease, and to communicate effectively by evaluating the feelings of others. From the beginning of time, all humans have used intuition or energy field evaluation to choose a lover or a friend and identify a political foe or supporter. We all "read" all the time, and if we are paying attention, we can use this information (consciously or subconsciously) to our advantage. It is the same process at work that helps us to avoid the street that feels "dangerous," know someone is going to call before they do, or to locate imbalances in the body.

Reiji is the ability to find imbalances in the body through intuition or guidance. In this protocol, your hands are guided to locations that will allow for optimal healing of the client. As this is an intuitive process, it is experienced very differently from person to person. It is important for the healer to know how they receive their intuition in order to be effective at this method of healing. The more aware you are of your own intuitive method, the more likely you are to notice cues. This is helpful both in healing protocols, and in everyday life.

Instructions

1. Stand or sit near the client and connect to the chi using Reiki.
2. Focus your attention on the client and set your intention to be guided to the priority area of healing.
3. Use your intuition and scan your senses for directions on where to place your hands. Notice how you are receiving the information. Do you hear directions telling you where to go? Do you feel a pull to a specific part of the body? Does a certain point on the body "light up" either literally or in your mind's

eye? Do you feel a sensation somewhere in your own body that might match up with an area of need on the client's body? Do you smell or taste something?

4. Use the information you receive and move your hands to the priority area for healing.
5. Allow the energy to flow to this area as long as necessary.
6. When the energy subsides, repeat the procedure for the next area requiring attention.
7. Continue this pattern until no other areas of the body call for attention.

Reiki Meridian Balance

After many years of working with clients, Valerie was looking for a simple way to directly balance the meridians using Reiki. By combining her knowledge of both Reiki and energy kinesiology, she created the Reiki meridian balance. With this protocol, Reiki is used at either the beginning or the end of the affected meridians. Muscle testing is used to direct the process. With an attunement to Reiki, a basic knowledge of meridians, and a little bit of muscle testing prowess, this meridian balance can be used anytime anywhere.

Instructions

1. Start with an indicator muscle that can lock and unlock. (See the muscle testing section of the "Tools" chapter.)
2. Check for energetic scrambling. (See the muscle testing section of the "Tools" chapter.)
3. Work with the client to set a positive, present-tense goal for the balance. (For example, "I climb stairs with ease" or "I am calm and relaxed in all situations.") Have the client state the goal while you test an indicator muscle. The muscle should unlock.

4. Determine how many meridians need Reiki in order to complete the balance. Say, "I am looking for the priority number of meridians to balance. One, two …" Test the indicator muscle after each number until there is a change in response. The number for which the indicator muscle changes is the number of meridians you will balance.

5. Now determine which meridians need Reiki and in which order. Say, "I am looking for the first priority meridian to balance." Then test the indicator muscle as you say the name of each meridian until there is a change in response. This is the first meridian. Continue doing this until you have the number of meridians found in the previous step.

6. Once you have found which meridians to balance, start with the first priority meridian. Test to see if you need to start at the beginning point of the meridian or the endpoint. Say, "I need to start at the endpoint." Then test the indicator muscle. If the response is a locked indicator, then you start at the endpoint. If not, test "I need to start at the beginning point." A locked indicator response means you start at the beginning point.

7. Test to see how far off the body you should hold your hands. Say "I am looking for the priority distance to hold my hands off the body." Then say "one inch," and test, then "two inches," and test, and so on, testing each measurement until there is an indicator change. The measurement where the indicator changes is the proper distance.

8. Now position your hands the determined distance over the determined meridian point. Use Reiki and allow chi to flow, with the intention that it flows through the specific meridian, clearing away any negativity, blockages, imbalances, etc.

9. When you feel the rise and fall of energy has subsided, or you feel the meridian is in balance, muscle test to make sure the correction is complete. Test "This meridian is complete." If the indicator locks on this statement, then proceed to the next step. If not, continue sending Reiki until you get a locked response to this statement.

10. Move on to the next meridian on your list and repeat steps 6 to 9.

11. Continue this process until you have balanced all the meridians found in step 4 and 5.
12. Have the client restate the goal and test the indicator muscle. The muscle should now lock. The balance is complete.

Reiki Spiral (Spiral Chakra Balancing)

There are many ways to balance the chakra system. As we described earlier, each chakra has different functions, aspects, and relationships to body systems. Depending on the person and the issue, one method may be more beneficial than another at a particular time. The spiral method is great for overall balancing. It can be used at the beginning of a traditional Reiki session, or it can be a standalone balance when specific chakra work is needed.

The spiral method gets its name from the way in which the hands move from point to point during the session.

<u>Instructions</u>

1. Starting with the heart chakra, place one hand a few inches above the chakra and the other at your side, palm facing up. Hold this position until there is a rise and fall of energy.
2. Move the hand that is over the chakra in a clockwise direction to the next chakra on the list below. The clockwise movement from one chakra to the next creates the spiral pattern. (See figure 22.)
3. Once number 12, the transpersonal point, is reached, the process is reversed. This time, move in a counterclockwise direction from one chakra or point to the next, tracing the spiral back in the opposite direction. It is not necessary to wait for the rise and fall of energy this time. Simply make contact with each chakra for a few seconds before moving on to the next one.
4. Finish with your hand above the heart chakra.

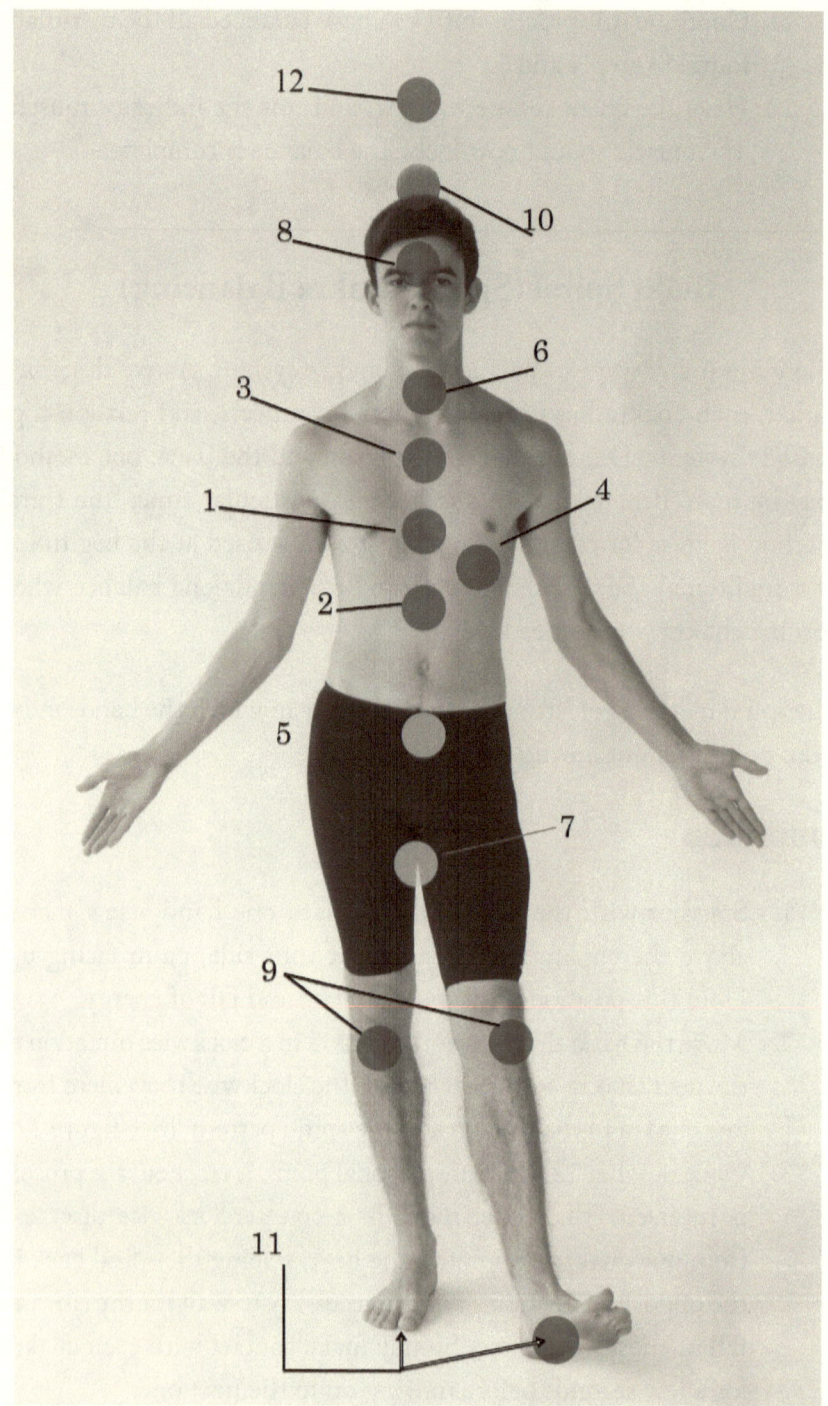

Figure 22: Reiki Spiral

Order for Reiki Spiral

1. **heart chakra** – center of the chest between breasts
2. **solar plexus chakra**– at the base of the sternum
3. **high heart point**– at the thymus, just below notch at the top of the sternum
4. **spleen point**– left side, near the seventh and eighth ribs
5. **sacral chakra**– two to three inches below navel
6. **throat chakra** – throat
7. **root chakra**– just below the pubic area
8. **third eye chakra** – middle of forehead
9. **knees** – one hand on top of each knee
10. **crown chakra**– top of the head
11. **feet** – one hand on the bottom of each foot
12. **transpersonal point**– six inches above the head

Balancing Chakras with Marmas

This simple but powerful chakra balancing approach involves the use of marmas and was developed by Marina.

When addressing imbalanced chakras, a hand is placed over the corresponding marma and held there until the chi balances. This approach technically does not open chakras directly, but helps to remove the blockage and restore the normal flow of chi. It is a very gentle approach that opens chakras slowly allowing your client to release blockages gradually, adjust to all the changes, and learn how to maintain strong, balanced chakras.

A note about marma names: For the purpose of this book, we have given marmas simplified English names. The traditional Indian names can be found in any marma therapy book. Please see the bibliography for suggestions.

Root Chakra

The root chakra can be balanced by putting your hands on two sets of marmas, inside the elbows and under the knees. It actually does not matter if you put your hands inside, under, or over the elbow or knee, simply make it a comfortable position. In either case, these marmas are very big and the chi from your hand goes far enough to reach the point.

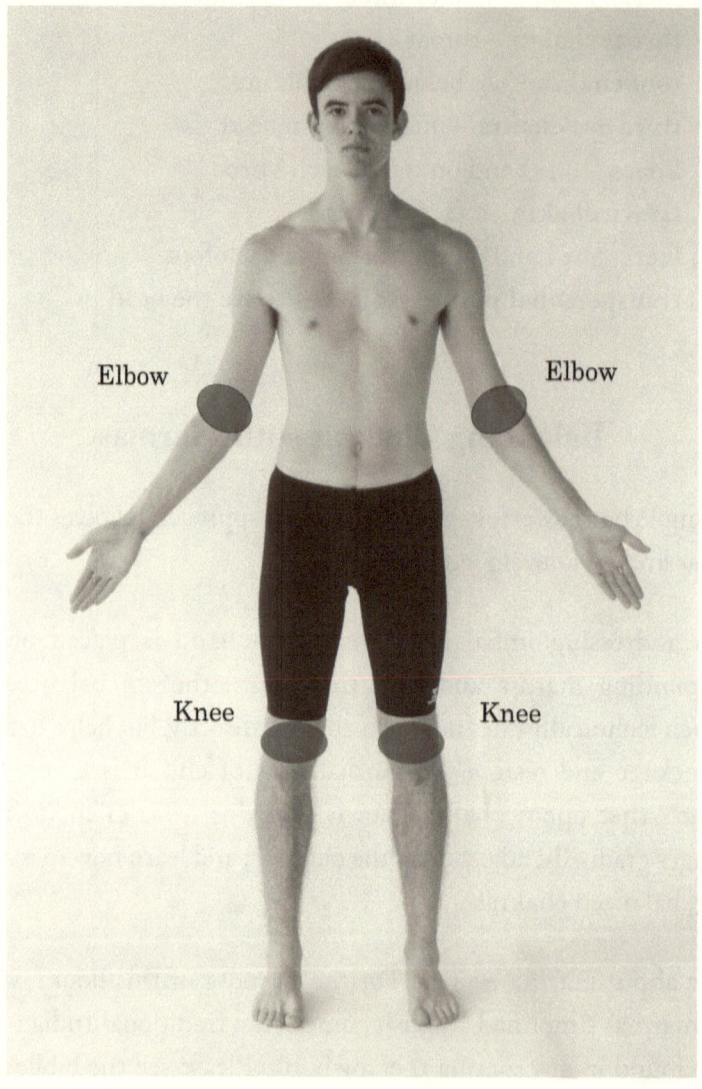

Figure 23: Root Chakra Balancing

<u>Use one of the following combinations:</u>

- right elbow and left elbow, then right knee and left knee
- right elbow and right knee, then left elbow and left knee

Marma points can assist with:

- bladder tone
- urinary dysfunction
- normal arm movement
- localized pain relief
- pancreatic dysfunction
- neuropathy
- tremors
- lymphedema
- carpal tunnel
- colon function
- expelling toxins
- releasing stagnant emotions
- irritable bowel syndrome
- any bowel inflammation
- menstrual cramps
- tennis elbow
- circulation
- arthritis
- low back pain
- vertigo
- asthma

Sacral Chakra

To open the sacral chakra, put your hands on the spleen marma and the left elbow. The spleen marma is located on the left side of the body, below the nipple, a few inches above the end of the ribcage. (In traditional Chinese medicine, this is a spleen acupuncture point.)

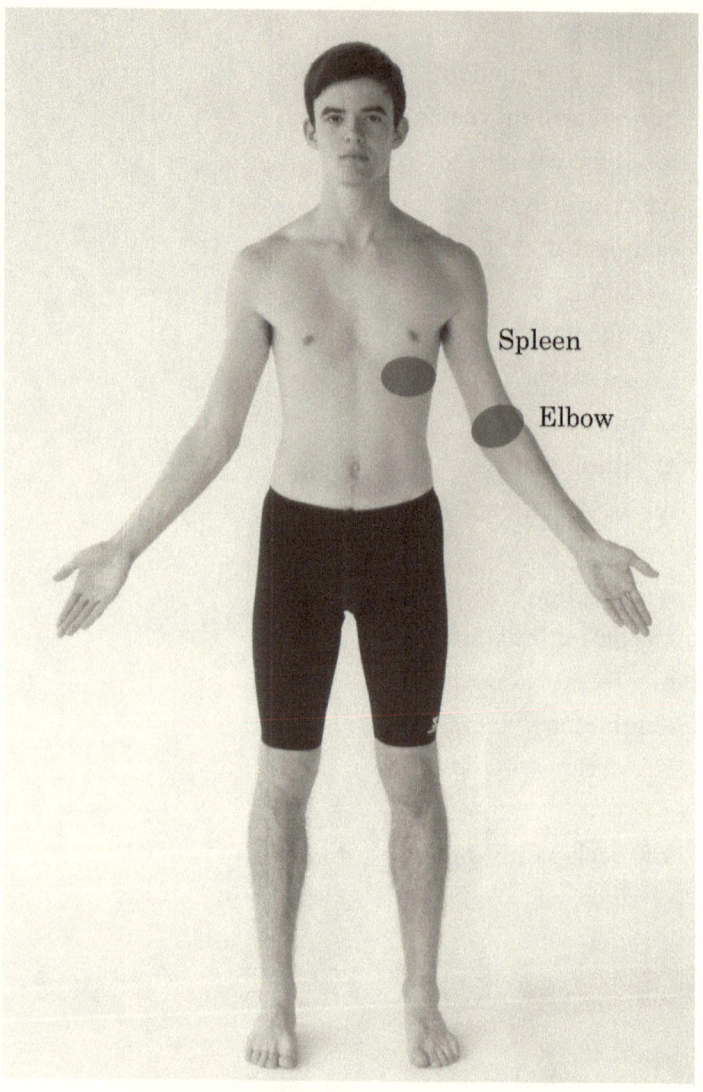

Spleen

Elbow

Figure 24: Sacral Chakra Balancing

Marma points can assist with:

- spleen function
- detoxification
- low immunity
- lymphatic circulation
- small intestine and
  colon function
- local pain
- anemia
- chronic fatigue syndrome
- diarrhea/constipation
- emotional turmoil

Solar Plexus Chakra

To open the solar plexus chakra, put your hand on the spleen marma located on the left side of the body, below the nipple, a few inches above the end of the ribcage. (In traditional Chinese medicine, this is a spleen acupuncture point.)

Next put one hand over the solar plexus. Hover the other hand about an inch above the belly button and make circular motions about six to seven inches wide.

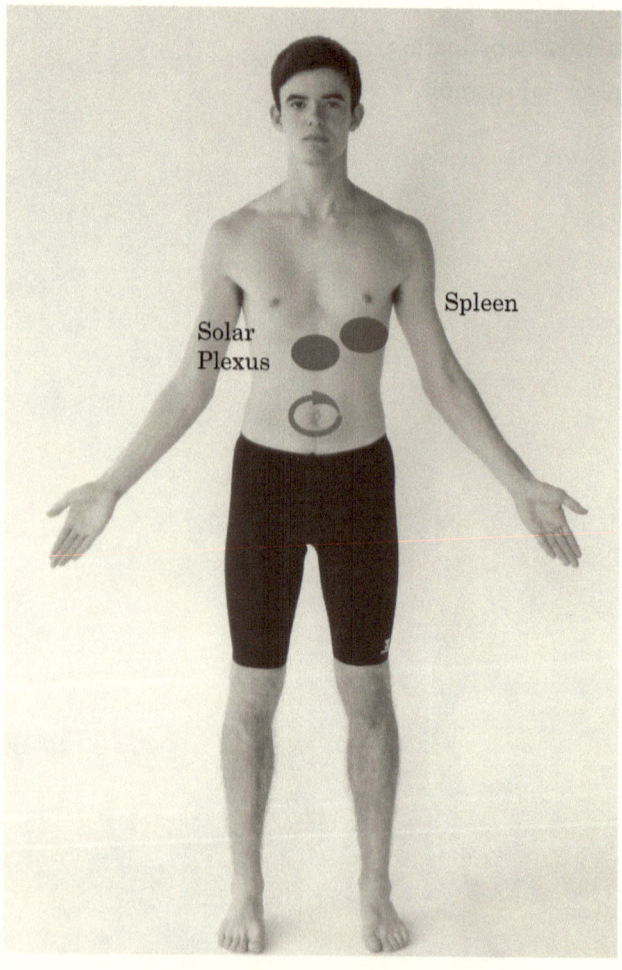

Figure 25: Solar Plexus Chakra Balancing

Marma points can assist with:

- spleen function
- detoxification
- low immunity
- lymphatic circulation
- small intestine and colon function
- local pain
- anemia
- chronic fatigue syndrome
- emotional turmoil
- liver dysfunction
- gall bladder dysfunction
- anorexia
- lactation
- abdominal pain
- digestion and absorption
- stomach function
- pancreas function
- constipation/diarrhea
- nausea/vomiting
- immune disorders

Heart Chakra

The heart chakra can be balanced by applying chi to the rib marmas located on both sides of the body and the ear marmas located immediately below the ears. (Cover the entire ear area with your palm.)

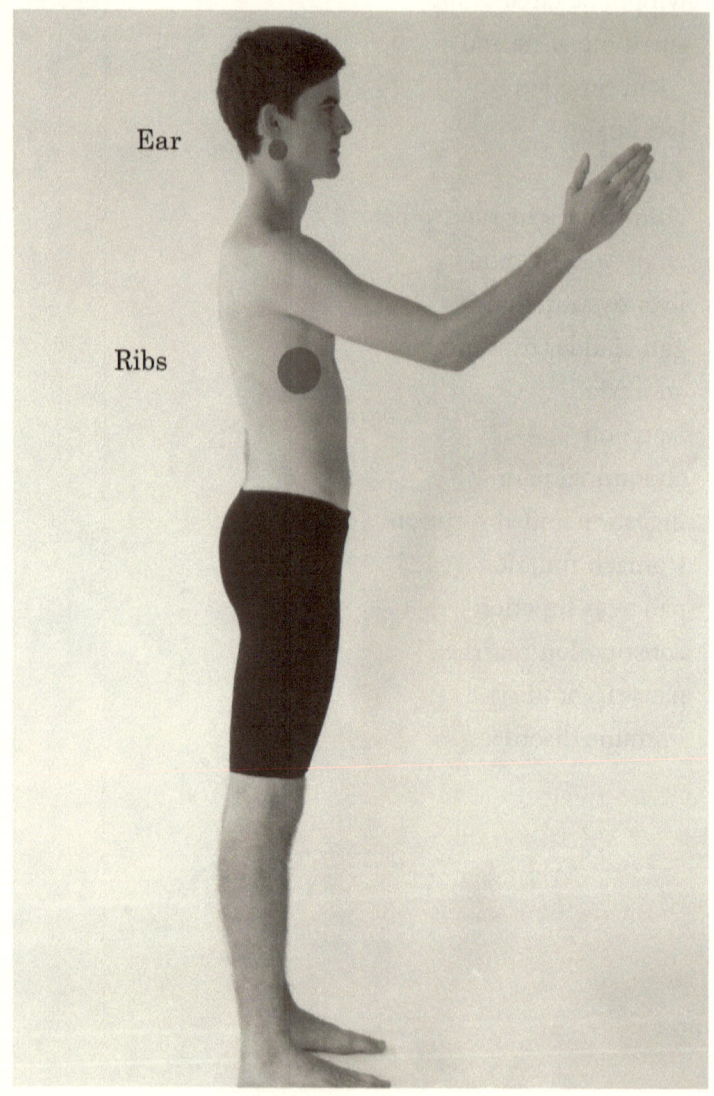

Figure 26: Heart Chakra Balancing

Use one of the following combinations:

- right ribs and right ear, then left ribs and left ear
- right ear and left ear, then both hands on right ribs and then both hands on left ribs

Marma points can assist with:

- flow of chi
- lung function
- asthma
- hiccups
- chronic cough
- chest pain
- intercostal pain
- liver pain
- spleen pain
- liver/spleen congestion
- kidney pain
- kidney stones
- abdominal pain
- Bell's palsy
- headaches and migraines
- kidney function
- ear disorders
- toothache
- vertigo
- blurry vision
- hyperactive mind
- ADHD
- stress and anxiety
- lower back pain
- TMJ pain

Throat Chakra

To open the throat chakra, put your hands over the shoulder marmas located on the top of the shoulder joint and over the navel marma, which is located on both sides of the navel.

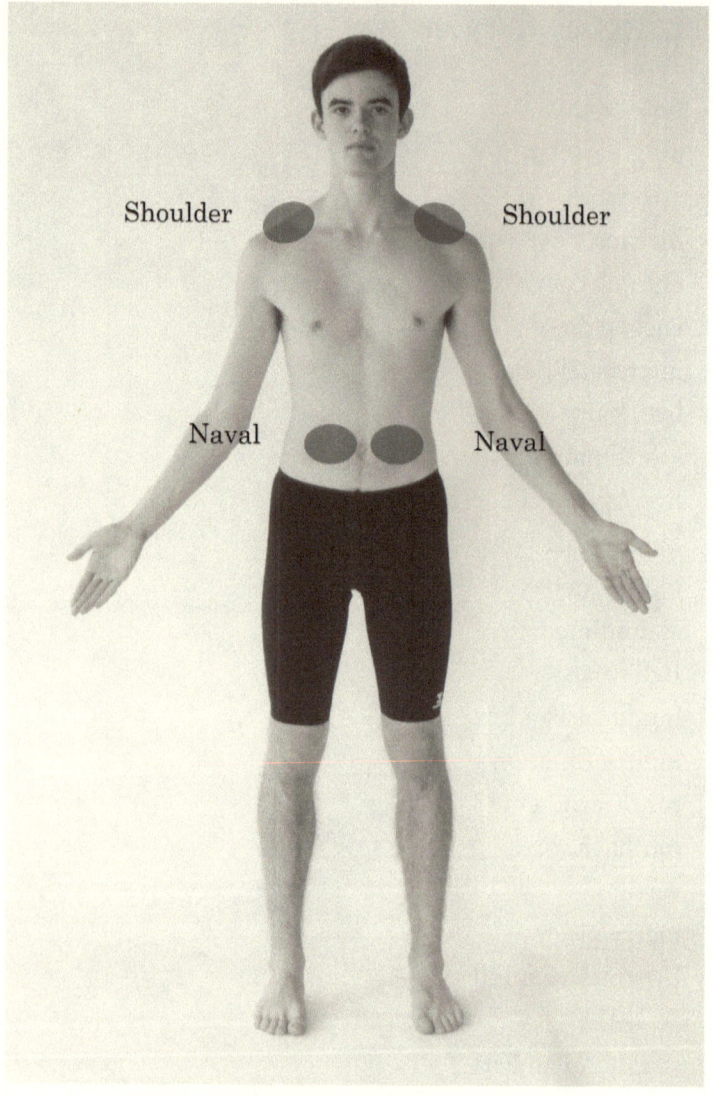

Figure 27: Throat Chakra Balancing

<u>Use one of the following combinations:</u>

- right shoulder and left shoulder, then right navel and left navel
- right shoulder and right navel, then left shoulder and left navel

Marma points can assist with:

- shoulder movement
- flow of chi
- shoulder pain
- frozen shoulder
- asthma
- bronchitis
- palpitation
- ringing in the ear
- earaches
- pancreatic dysfunction
- stress
- fatigue
- liver pain
- spleen pain
- liver/spleen congestion
- kidney pain
- kidney stones
- abdominal pain

Third Eye Chakra

The third eye chakra can be opened by putting the hands over the temple marmas (located just in front of the ear on both sides of the head), the collarbone marma (in the middle of the collarbone), and the groin marma(located in the lower part of abdomen).

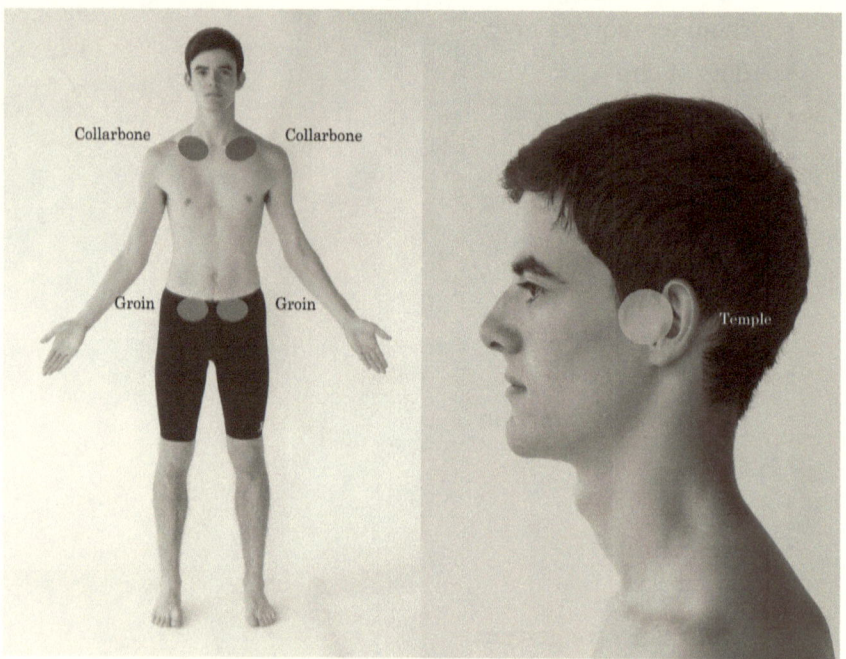

Figure 28: Third Eye Chakra Balancing

Use the following combination:

- right and left temple, then right collarbone and right groin; then left collarbone and left groin

Marma points can assist with:

- headaches and migraines
- stomach pain
- colon function
- ear, eye, teeth, and face function
- speech
- calming the mind
- reproductive organs
- digestion

Crown Chakra

The crown chakra balances beautifully using the hand marmas, located in the middle of the palm, and the foot marmas, located in the arch of the foot.

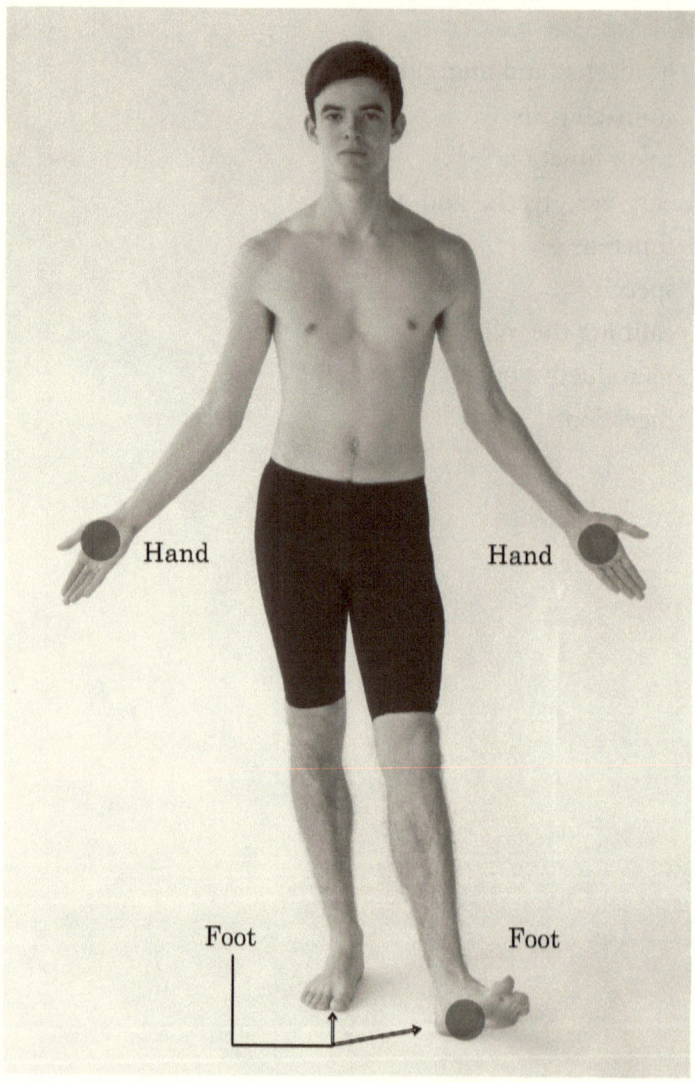

Figure 29: Crown Chakra Balancing

<u>Use one of the following combinations:</u>

- right hand and left hand, then right foot and left foot
- right hand and right foot, then left hand and left foot

Marma points can assist with:

- balancing heart and mind
- harmonizing emotions
- lowering stress
- relieving emotional disturbance
- relieving headaches
- helping with balance
- calming the mind

CLOSING PROTOCOLS

Methods for harmonizing, cleaning and closing
the energy field at the end of a session

Chakra Balancing Protocols

In the following protocols, the chakras are balanced to be in harmony with one another. The methods are different only in the order in which the chakras are addressed. In each one, the hands are placed over two chakras simultaneously and held there until the chi quiets and equalizes. In our experience, it is highly beneficial to close a Reiki session with one of these protocols.

Basic Ayurvedic Balance

The approach here is to balance each chakra against the crown chakra.

Instructions

1. Put one hand over the crown chakra and leave it there for the remainder of the balance.
2. Put the other hand over each of the following chakras in order. Hold each position until the chi quiets and equalizes.
   - root chakra
   - sacral chakra
   - solar plexus chakra
   - heart chakra
   - throat chakra
   - third eye chakra

Basic Symmetry Balance

In this protocol, the chakras are balanced in pairs.

Instructions

Place one hand on each chakra in the pairs below, and hold until the chi quiets and equalizes. Balance the chakras in the following order:

1. crown – root
2. third eye – sacral
3. throat – sacral
4. heart – solar plexus

Chakra Emotional Balancing

This protocol is used when the chakras need to release a lot of negative emotions. Use this if you have applied any mental and emotional protocols during the session.

Instructions

1. Put one hand over the third eye chakra and leave it there for the remainder of the balance.
2. Put the other hand over each of the following chakras in order. Hold each position until the chi quiets and equalizes.
   - root chakra
   - sacral chakra
   - solar plexus chakra
   - heart chakra
   - throat chakra
   - crown chakra

Spirit-Mind Chakra Balancing

Use this protocol when the reconnection among mind, spirit, and emotions is required.

Instructions

1. With one hand, touch the crown and third eye chakras at the same time. Leave this hand here for the remainder of the balance.
2. Put the other hand over each of the following chakras in order. Hold each position until the chi quiets and equalizes.
   * root chakra
   * sacral chakra
   * solar plexus chakra
   * heart chakra
   * throat chakra

Traditional Japanese Protocols

The following protocols are used at the end of a session and are intended to help rid the body of toxic energies. They are thought to stimulate blood flow and therefore hasten healing to imbalanced areas.

Ketsueki Koukan Ho: Blood Cleansing

This protocol is also called the Reiki finish or nerve stroke as taught by Hawayo Takata in the West. It is thought to rid the body of toxins and stagnant energy.

Instructions

1. With the client lying face down, stand so that your non-dominant hand is near the head. (The non-dominant hand is the hand through which you tend to sense less energy. The dominant hand is the one you would tend to perform Reiki with and feel the energy more powerfully.)
2. Place the non-dominant hand lightly at the top of the spine near the base of the skull.
3. Place the dominant hand, palm flat, just below the other hand across the top of the spine.
4. Stroke gently *downward* with the dominant hand, from the top of the spine to the base of the spine. This can be done directly on the body with gentle pressure or in the energy field within three inches of the body. When you reach the base of the spine, lift your hand up off the body and use an arcing motion (like a rainbow) to return your hand to the starting position at the top of the spine. Repeat this stroking motion ten to fifteen times.
5. Place one hand at the top of the spine and the other at the base of the spine and hold this position until the energy is equal in both directions.

Zenshin Koketsu Ho: Full Body Blood Cleansing

This protocol is another version of blood cleansing used to rid the body of toxins and stagnant energy.

Instructions

1. Treat the head, chest, and abdomen (lungs, heart, stomach, and intestines) using the traditional hand positions.
2. With the client lying either face up or face down, stroke gently down each arm from the shoulder to the tips of the fingers. This

can be done directly on the body with gentle pressure or in the energy field within three inches of the body. When you reach the fingertips, lift your hand up off the body and use an arcing motion (like a rainbow) to return your hand to the starting position at the shoulder. Repeat this stroking motion ten to fifteen times.

3. Starting at the outside of the hips, stroke down each leg from the hip to the tips of the toes. Again, this can be done directly on the body with gentle pressure or in the energy field within three inches of the body. When you reach the tips of the toes, lift your hand up off the body and use an arcing motion to return your hand to the starting position at the hip. Repeat this stroking motion ten to fifteen times.

APPENDIX

Simple Meditation

Though designed to be used with the emotional release protocol, this simple meditation can be used at any time to help your client relax.

Instructions

Read each statement below in a calm and soothing voice. Make sure to pause at least five seconds after each phrase to give your client a chance to do what you have suggested.

> Let's start the meditation with the deep breath.
> Become aware of your body.
> Become aware of your feet.
> Become aware of your legs.
> Become aware of your torso.
> Become aware of your arms.
> Become aware of your hands.
> Become aware of your shoulders.
> Become aware of your neck.
> Become aware of your head.
> Become aware of your breath.

You can now either continue with the chosen protocol or allow the client to simply breathe and relax for a while before ending the meditation.

GLOSSARY

Acupuncture – A therapy used to stimulate energy flow and balance meridians by applying needles to specific points on the human body called acupuncture points.

Acupuncture Points – Specific points along the meridians that are used to stimulate energy flow.

Acute Protocols – Reiki protocols that are used in specific circumstances for acute emotional or energetic disturbances: chakra shooting, chakra spreading, tapping (Uchi-te Chiyo-ho), and pulsing (Oshi-te Chiryo-ho).

Alternative Hand Position Protocol – A sequence of hand positions developed by Marina Lando in 2010, out of a desire for faster and more significant results for her clients. They are highly effective, easy on the client, and more comfortable for the practitioner than the basic hand positions.

Aromatherapist – A practitioner professionally trained in the art of aromatherapy.

Aromatherapy – The art of the application of essential oils for emotional, spiritual, and physical healing.

Attunement – The process by which Reiki students are connected to the flow of chi from the universe.

Ayurveda – A five-thousand-year-old wellness system from India with an extensive understanding of a wide range of subjects from prevention and balancing to surgery, herbal medicine, and psychology. It is still used by many doctors in India, Europe, and America. According to Ayurveda, there is no separation between the physical and energetic body. Mind, spirit, and body affect each other on a constant basis.

Base Chakra – See root chakra.

Basic Ayurvedic Chakra Balancing – An approach used to balance each chakra against the crown chakra.

Basic Hand Positions – Hand positions typically taught in Reiki 1 that make it easy for beginners and advanced practitioners alike to perform a very beneficial healing session. Each hand position stimulates specific meridians, chakras, marmas, etc.

Basic Symmetry Balancing – A chakra balance that balances the chakras in pairs.

Bliss Body – The soul or body of light (Ayurveda).

Blockage – A mental, emotional, spiritual, or physical obstacle that prevents the flow of energy.

Blood Cleansing – Also called the Reiki finish or nerve stroke as taught by Hawayo Takata in the West. It is thought to rid the body of toxins and stagnant energy.

Body Scanning – A method of detecting energy imbalances by moving the hand over the body and noting changes in the feel of the energy.

Breath Body – According to Ayurveda, this is the energy that holds together the physical body.

Byosan Reikan-Ho – This is an original technique for body scanning from Master Usui, which can be used either as self-treatment or to help others. The words *Byosan Reikan* describe the energy of an imbalance as detected by the hands. Byosan Reikan literally means energy sensation of sickness (imbalance/disease). Byo means disease or sickness, and San means before, ahead, previous, future, or precedence. Rei means energy, soul, or spirit, and kan means emotion, feeling, or sensation.

Chakras – Energy vortexes that reflect a person's physical, mental, spiritual, and emotional state. They have their roots in the spine and grow through the body toward the front. There are seven chakras: root (or base), sacral, solar plexus (or power), heart, throat, third eye, and crown. Each of these chakras is associated with a specific function and provides the energy and information exchange among all living organisms and between living organism and environment. When the chakras are open, there is a balance. Blockages in the chakras can cause disturbances in all levels of consciousness.

Chakra Balancing – Removing blockages and toxic emotions from the chakras in order to help restore natural energy flow to the body.

Chakra Emotional Balancing – A method of balancing the chakras that uses the third eye chakra, paired with each of the other chakras in order, to release negative emotions.

Chakra Shooting – A method used to add additional energy to closed chakras. It is used when most of the chakras are closed as a result of prolonged, continued stress.

Chakra Spreading – A method of chakra balancing where the hands are used to spread the energy of the chakras outward. It is used as soon as possible after a major traumatic event, such as the death of a friend or family member, an accident, major surgery, or divorce, in order to minimize the impact of imbalanced energy.

Chi – Life-force energy.

Closing Protocols – Balancing processes used to close a Reiki session.

Crown Chakra – An energy vortex located at the top of the head.

Distant Symbol – Also called the third symbol, this is one of the three symbols to which Reiki students are attuned in Reiki level 2.

Earth Element – One of the five elements from Chinese Five Element Theory related to the emotions of empathy and sympathy.

Earth Meridians – The meridians associated with the earth element (i.e., stomach meridian and spleen meridian).

Emotional Release Protocol – A process used to release negative emotions that is done by "unlocking" the emotional points on the forehead, just above the center of the eyebrows.

Emotional Symbol – Also called the second symbol, this is one of the three symbols to which Reiki students are attuned in Reiki level 2.

Energy Healing – The process of removing energetic blockages, toxic emotions, and stress patterns in order to help the body's energy (chi, prana, qi, ki) flow freely and aid the body in healing itself.

Evaluation – The process by which the practitioner gathers information about the client and his energy patterns in order to plan the session.

Fire Element – One of the five elements from Chinese Five Element Theory related to the emotions of joy, love, and hate.

Fire Meridians – The meridians associated with the fire element (i.e., small intestine meridian, heart meridian, triple warmer meridian, and circulation-sex meridian).

Focused Healing – See Byosan Reikan-Ho.

Heart Chakra – An energy vortex located at the center of the chest.

Horary Cycle – The twenty-four hour cycle of energy flow through the meridians. Each meridian, and its associated organ, has a two hour period where it is at its maximum energy and activity.

Human Energy Field – A dynamic field of energy that surrounds and supports the human body. This energy field, like the physical body, is comprised of many individual systems that work together to maintain our health. The physical body and the energy field feed, support, and affect one another. In order for the whole person to be healthy and balanced, there must be harmony between the energetic and the physical.

Intuitive Healing – See Reiji.

Ketsueki Koukan Ho – See blood cleansing.

Ki – See chi.

Kinesiology – 1.) The science and study of muscle movement. 2.) The science and art of muscle testing for energy imbalances and correcting them. (This second definition applies to kinesiology as used in this book.)

Koshas – Also known as "bodies." These are the levels of self that make up a whole person. Energy flows through each one, connecting them and helping us maintain our vitality. Ayurveda recognizes five koshas: bliss body, wisdom body, mental body, breath body, and the physical or food body.

Marmas – Areas on the body that assist the free exchange of chi and information between the physical and energy bodies and can be used to balance physical and emotional disturbances. Many marma point locations correspond directly with the location of acupuncture points from traditional Chinese medicine. Though marmas are sometimes called "minor chakras "or "secondary chakras," marmas and chakras are actually very different.

Master Symbol – Also called the fourth symbol, this is the final symbol to which Reiki students are attuned at the master level.

Mental and Emotional Reiki Protocol – A process used to calm the mind and help the body release blockages that are being held by stuck emotions.

Mental Body – According to Ayurveda, this body represents personhood.

Meridian Cycle – See horary cycle.

Meridians – Energy lines or highways that carry vital energy to all parts of the body. They feed the muscles and organs and provide the energy that keeps us balanced and healthy. Disruption in the flow of the meridians can lead to imbalance and stress on the physical, mental, emotional, or spiritual levels.

Metal Element – One of the five elements from Chinese Five Element Theory related to the emotions of grief, guilt, and regret.

Metal Meridians – The meridians associated with the metal element (i.e., large intestine meridian and lung meridian).

Muscle Testing – A method of biofeedback that involves applying gentle pressure against a muscle's range of motion and observing its behavior. The muscle's responses give the tester information about the energy flow in the body (i.e., how the body responds to different stimuli).

Nadis – Channels that move the chi energy through the body. A total of 72,000 nadis branch from the seventh chakra (crown chakra) and encompass the whole body. There are fourteen principal nadis.

Ochi-te Chiryo-ho (Pulsing) – A specific hand movement used to encourage energy flow and stimulate circulation by drawing energy and awareness to an area of the body.

Past Life Regression Protocol – A process that helps to release blockages that may have been acquired in previous lives so our life lessons may be seen more clearly.

Pendulum – An ancient tool used to divine information and determine the state of the chakras. It is comprised of a small piece of wood, metal, stone, or other natural material attached at the end of a string or a chain.

Physical or Food Body – According to Ayurveda, this is the actual physical body or physical self.

Power Chakra – See solar plexus chakra.

Power Symbol – Also called the first symbol, this is one of the three symbols to which Reiki students are attuned in Reiki level 2.

Prana – See chi.

Pulsing – See Ochi-te Chiryo-ho.

Qi – See chi.

Qigong – ("Life-Energy Cultivation") A practice used to cultivate and balance chi by aligning the body, breath, and mind.

Reiki – A system of natural healing developed by Mikao Usui. It involves applying chi (prana, ki, qi) to the body in order to remove blockages and balance the chi flow.

Reiki Master – A Reiki practitioner who has achieved the highest level of Reiki attunements.

Reiki Meridian Balance – An energy balancing process developed by Valerie Remhoff where muscle testing is used to determine which meridians are involved, and Reiki is then used to send chi to either the beginning or endpoint of those meridians in order to achieve balance.

Reiki Practitioner – A person professionally trained in Reiki.

Reiki Protocol – A process or technique for administering healing energy that involves the use of Reiki.

Reiki Session – A period of time devoted to healing where Reiki is utilized.

Reiki Spiral – A process for balancing the chakra system where each chakra is given energy in a specific sequence that takes the shape of a spiral.

Reiki Symbols – Specific patterns of lines that are traditionally only given to students with second degree Reiki training and above. They help the Reiki practitioner to achieve different goals during a Reiki session.

Reiji – The ability to find imbalances in the body through intuition or guidance.

Root Chakra – An energy vortex originating at the base of the spine. (Also called base chakra.)

Sacral Chakra – An energy vortex located at the lower part of the abdomen.

Self-Care Reiki – The application of Reiki to oneself.

Solar Plexus Chakra – An energy vortex located at the solar plexus. (Also called the power chakra.)

Spirit-Mind Chakra Balancing – A process of chakra balancing that is used when the reconnection among mind, spirit, and emotions is required.

Stress Release Protocol – A process of relieving stress and emotional turmoil by placing the hands over emotional points on the forehead.

Tapping – See Uchi-te Chiyo-ho.

Third Eye Chakra – An energy vortex located between eyebrows.

Throat Chakra – An energy vortex located at the throat.

Touch for Health – A system of natural healthcare, developed by Dr. John Thie. Muscle testing is utilized along with simple correction methods to help balance the body's energy and relieve stress and tension.

Traditional Chinese Medicine – A system of medicine that originated in China thousands of years ago that includes the use of herbal medicines and various mind and body practices.

Transpersonal Point – An energy point that is located six inches above the head.

Uchi-te Chiyo-ho – The use of a tapping hand motion on the energy field to relieve stress and tension, improve circulation, and relieve congestion.

Water Element – One of the five elements from Chinese Five Element Theory related to the emotions of fear and anxiety.

Water Meridians – The meridians associated with the water element (i.e., bladder meridian and kidney meridian).

Wisdom Body – According to Ayurveda, this is the manifestation of the intellect.

Wood Element – One of the five elements from Chinese Five Element Theory related to the emotions of anger and resentment.

Wood Meridians – The meridians associated with the wood element (i.e., gall bladder meridian and liver meridian).

Yang – According to Chinese philosophy, this is male, active energy.

Yin – According to Chinese philosophy, this is female, passive energy.

Zenshin Koketsu Ho (full body blood cleansing) – A process where the energy field is brushed with the hand in a specific pattern in order to rid the body of toxins and stagnant energy.

BIBLIOGRAPHY

- Anodea, Judith. *Wheels of Life*. St. Paul, MN: Llewellyn Publications, 2004.
- Cohen, Kenneth. *The Way of Qi Gong*. New York: Ballantine Books, 1997.
- Cross, John. *Acupuncture and the Chakra Energy System*. Berkley, CA: North Atlantic Books, 2008.
- Eden, Donna. *Energy Medicine*. New York: Penguin, 2008.
- Frawley, David, Subbash Ranade and Avinsh Lele. *Ayurveda and Marma Therapy*. Twin Lake, WI: Lotus Press, 2009.
- Lad, Vasant and Anisha Durve. *Marma Points of Ayurveda*. Albuquerque, NM: The Ayurvedic Press, 2008.
- Lubek, Walter, Frank Arjava Petter and William Lee Rand. *The Spirit of Reiki*. Twin Lake, WI: Lotus Press, 2003.
- Morris, P. L., B. Raphael, and R. G. Robinson. "Clinical Depression Is Associated with Impaired Recovery from Stroke." *The Medical Journal of Australia* 157, vol. 4 (1992): 239–242.
- Petter, Frank Arjava, Tadao Yamaguchi, Chujiro Hayashi. *The Hayashi Reiki Manual*. Twin Lake, WI: Lotus Press, 2003.
- Petter, Frank Arjava. *Reiki Fire*. Twin Lake, WI: Lotus Press, 2005.
- Rand, William Lee. *Reiki: The Healing Touch First and Second Degree Manual*. Southfield, MI: Vision Publications, 2005.
- Tedeschi, Mark. *Essential Anatomy for Healing and Marshal Arts*. Boston: Whitehill, 2008.

- Thie, John F., and Matthew Thie. *Touch for Health. The Complete Edition: A Practical Guide to Natural Health with Acupressure Touch and Massage.* Camarillo, CA: DeVorss Publications, 2005.
- Tirtha, Swami Sadashiva. *The Ayurveda Encyclopedia.* Unadilla, NY: Ayurveda Holistic Center Press, 2007.
- Yamaguchi, Tadao. *Light on the Origins of Reiki.* Twin Lake, WI: Lotus Press, 2007.
- Yang, Jwing-Ming. "The Eight Extraordinary Qi Vessels." Acupuncture.com. Accessed March 24, 2014. http://www.acupuncture.com/qigong_tuina/eightextra.htm.

INDEX

ABOUT THE AUTHORS

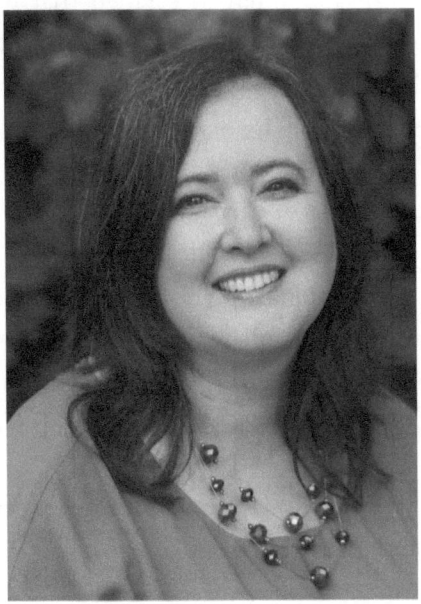

Marina Lando

MS, Reiki master teacher, aromatherapist (MarinaLando.me)

For as long as she can remember, Marina has been passionate about making people well. She was first introduced to natural healing by her grandmother at about the age of seven. Marina's grandmother would take her to a forest or a meadow near her home and show her what to collect, how to find plants, how they smelled and felt, and how to use them. The family cupboard always smelled of dried flowers, and linden tea is still Marina's first choice for a fever. When Marina had any pain, her grandmother would put her hand over Marina's body and the heat of her hands would soothe away the discomfort. Nobody called it Reiki, medical qigong, or any other exotic name. Marina just knew that her grandma was magic, and she wanted to be like her.

At the age of nine, Marina discovered the *Children's Encyclopedia of Chemistry* and read it cover to cover. She was amazed by the possibilities of mixing together chemicals and making drugs to cure diseases. At the same time, she was disappointed. It seemed that in many situations, plants that her grandmother gathered every year provided just as much healing opportunity without as much hassle. So she did not become a chemist or a pharmacist, but she married a chemist (just in case).

Circumstances led Marina to earn master's degrees in both computer science and economics. Later in life, she learned Reiki, Ayurveda, and aromatherapy professionally. She started her healing practice in 2007 and expanded into the full-service healing center Harmony Life (HarmonyLifeCary.com) in 2011. Marina continues to study and expand her knowledge, as there is always so much more to learn.

Marina lives in Cary, North Carolina, with her husband and son. She is a martial artist and an avid knitter.

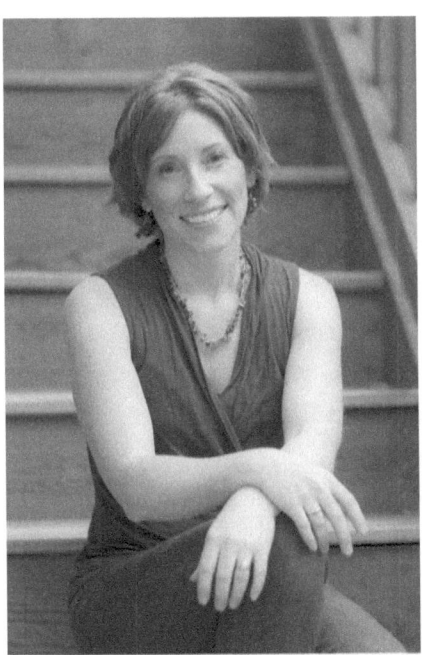

Valerie Remhoff

BA, Reiki master teacher, IKC certified Touch for Health instructor/consultant.

Valerie has always seen and worked with energy. From the time she was a little girl, she instinctively knew what to do to make someone feel better. The colors she saw around people were a normal part of life for her, and until someone told her that she was seeing auras, she thought everyone saw what she did!

Not knowing how best to make use of her natural talents, Valerie continued to develop them while pursuing other interests. She attained a bachelor's degree in environmental science from Rollins College in just three years, and shortly thereafter began a career in software engineering. It wasn't until her sister became very sick that Valerie's path became clear. After exhausting all the treatment options of conventional medicine, her sister's health was still declining. In search of another option, she began seeing a holistic practitioner. The change was amazing.

Through chiropractic, clinical kinesiology, nutrition, acupuncture, and other energy-balancing methods, she was able to reach a level of wellness that conventional medicine had found impossible to facilitate. Valerie was fascinated by the scientific and intuitive methodologies used in her sister's care and was astounded by her miraculous recovery. This experience inspired Valerie and set her on the path to becoming a holistic practitioner.

In 2005, Valerie left her career in software engineering and started practicing kinesiology and Reiki. She has never looked back. She is passionate about what she does and is honored to be helping others. She hopes to inspire more people to learn about natural healing methods and feel more empowered in their own health care.

Valerie lives in Holly Springs, North Carolina with her husband and their three boys, who are the sunshine of her life.

www.butterflyholistics.com